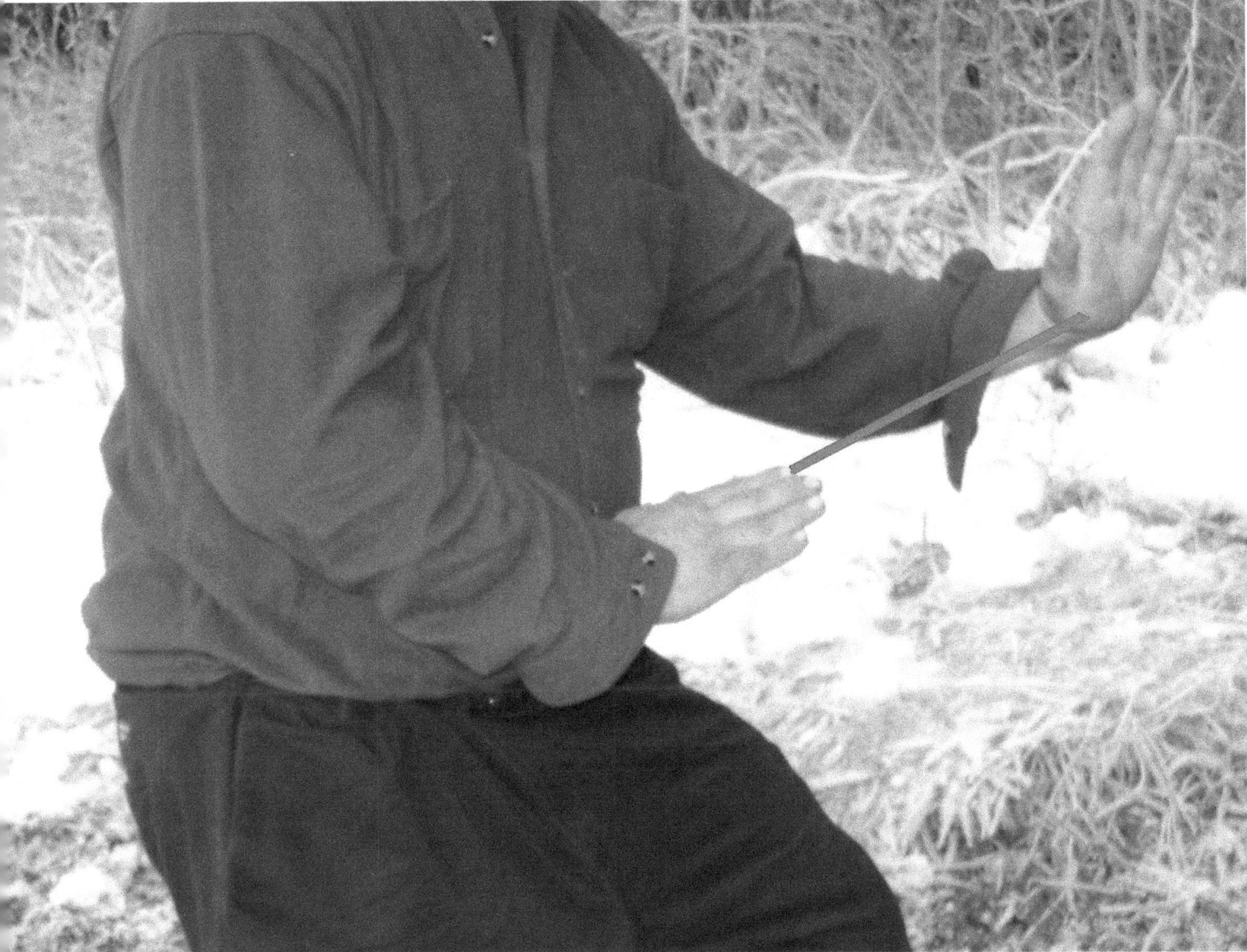

Axe Hand;

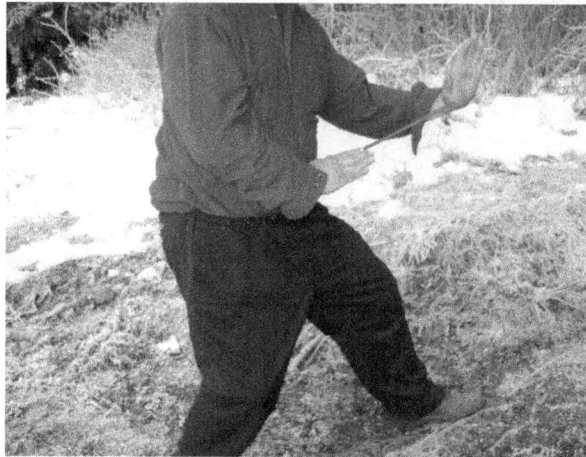

Hsing-i & Internal Strength Workout

Greg W. Hayes

Gregory W. Hayes
P.O. Box 22835
Juneau, AK 99802

This book is one part of training in Hsing-i and internal energy. Before beginning any training one should consult with their health care professional (N.D., Acupuncturist and/or M.D.).

The following, is for informational purposes only, and is in no way to be interpreted as diagnosis, treatment, or to take the place of training; it is best be used, by those already trained, to augment there knowledge base. All of the methods listed have been used by the author and students, but they are not appropriate for everyone.

A competent teacher is a student's best mirror and hope of focus. This book will help. It teaches how to feel Qi, not eye-based visualization. Sensing-seeing is done with your gut (Lower Dan Tien), hands, feet etc. Training is individually based and free of the limitations of different languages, religion, or culture; since ones own experience is utilized to learn to recognize previously felt sensations of positive and negative Qi. The 'Shared Lived Experience' and essences are the means of communication, and development. This eliminates the extra step of translation.

Qigong is based on meditative martial Northern Shaolin Buddhist methods, Internal Iron Shirt and Internal Iron Palm in the Wide Circle of Kung Fu of Joseph Greenstein (The Might Atom of Ripley's and Guinness Book of World Records. Hsing-i was studied under Grandmaster Wong Jack (Chia) Man of San Francisco Jing Mo (the first person to complete all of the Northern Shaolin studies since World War II). Sifu Wong's direct lineage can be traced to the Ching soldiers burning of Honan Shaolin Temple 1732 AD., when Monk Chi Yuan escaped and went to Shantung province. Sifu Hayes has taught Hsing-i, Shaolin, Tai Chi and Qigong at: the Yoga Den (Rainforest Yoga), in Juneau from 1991-1998; Juneau Public School's Community Schools, from 1991-2005; private lessons in Juneau, since 1995.

Table of Contents

INTRODUCTION

This training regimen is based on various focuses of physical fitness, internal strength, meditation, forms, drills and exercises. Origins range from: propriety traditional sets, general domain traditional internal sets, a general styles set, free form internal calisthenics (Chi Kung, Nei Gong and Wei Gong), Shaolin Buddhist meditation, fighting coaches, healers and old folk's drills.

The methods and techniques come from a number of schools of Internal Martial Arts; that are compatible with each other. None of these varied schools have ever physically warred directly with each other. This book does not contain any internal methods that I have learned that I know are from schools with historic military conflicts, or fundamental philosophical discrepancies. This avoids a chop-suey approach of using methods independent of their tenets, lacking a cohesive and qualitative growth.

There is no faster way to build up the body overall, than chopping or splitting wood since the entire body gets into the swing of things. Axing tones and strengthens the muscles, ligaments, and connective tissues with fluid whipped motions; that are well anchored, focused and coordinated. Axers are a jaded, hardy and tough lot; that are well rounded.

Axe Hand is usually referred to as the element metal, and is the primary set that Hsing-i's San ti static stance is used for Chi Kung (Qi Gong), similar to the Standing Pole (Embrace the Moon) exercise is used for Tai Chi and Bei Shaolin (Northern). Hsing-I uses the second row of knuckles, as a wedge.

In the past, only those who had reached the level of Abbots were taught Hsing-i.

This book makes no attempt to contain all of the theories, history and segregated school dogmas of Hsing-i. The reader should see what helps them in their practice, and in their understanding and use it based upon their own results. This is not the official dogma of any particular teacher or school, but a collection of practical aids to training. Those with different back grounds will experience different results.

This commonality gives credit to traditional and other training methods. In the monastic and spiritual perspective, this teaches what is in common, and does not emphasize the differences. Because it does not have the attachments of form and specific uses, it becomes timeless and transcendent.

Internal Martial Arts can be moving meditation. One can use this as a mirror to see oneself. For some, Internal Martial Arts are only for healing and show so they appear choreographing forms as a ballerina. They are pretty to watch but fail in a fight. Following others in a spoon-fed manner can be the actions of a parrot.

This book is not for those who want to be told **what** to think, but rather **how** to think using other consciousnesses. Training methods can tune sensitivities and perceptions for a new personal knowledge and power. This is not for memorizing official school lines but rather it is for those who want to have a deeper understanding based on their own feeling and insight gained by training. One does not have to believe in something if they can see it or feel it. The merits of a theory alone are used, not who said them, or what school they belong to.

This is for independent free thinkers who can benefit from training themselves, with what they have learned. A teacher shows something new, but is not required to hold your hand while you practice it.

The emphasis is on developing internal energies, rather than the forms. What is more important, is not the differences but what is in common with many internal practices. A karateka can have many forms but still use the same basic energy of tensing the muscles on impact and relying on momentum. Some kung fu trainers are no different.

This book is a tool not a bible, use what works. Everything has been used with positive results, by my self and my students.

Physics can explain light as a particle, and it can explain it as a wave. So is light one or the other? That is not the main concern. Be able to see something **through** any theory not **by** a theory. There is understanding in both models, and there is more to understanding than models.

When one totally accepts any theory, they have stopped thinking on their own, and are only memorizing what to think, rather than thinking themselves. This is not to say everyone has to reinvent the wheel on their own, but not to stop at the last invention

It is usually easier to flow Chi (Qi) through healthy muscle tissue, so weight training is used; not to build muscle bulk, but to tone the tissue. This type of training is not classical weight training in that the push is started in the Lower Dan Tien and moves to the arm or leg muscle. Normally, for most people, the only emphasis is in the contraction of only the immediate muscle between the joint that is moving.

Strenuous exercise is complimented with the stretches so as to minimize the effects of over pumping and stiff rigid muscles.
This integrates full body movement and energies so the body can respond flowingly and evenly to transmit combined power of all the parts involved.

Internal energy can be developed in many methods. For preliminary internal toning of the abdominal area and internal organ area of the body, one may use hundreds of pushups, sit-ups and meditation; to bring the Qi flow to a high enough level to proceed to higher levels of Qi Gong, Internal Iron Shirt and Internal Iron Palm. Others methods attain a strong internal energy flow through months doing Grand or Small Circulation Qi Gong or Iron Shirt Qi Gong Massage and beating.

Using the techniques in this book will strengthen internal energy so it is fit for combat, and use in everyday life. Qi will be used and felt like any other tool. This also lays the foundation for Iron Shirt, Cotton Belly, Golden Bell and Internal Iron Palm.

I have demonstrated Cotton Belly to many karate schools, weight lifters and boxers in California and Alaska, and no one can hurt my abdominal area with any combination of blows or kicks.

Internal Striking has been demonstrated by me likewise, by having a soft material such as a four inch thick phone book placed over a volunteer, who will feel the strike through the material. No one has asked for more force.

Before studying martial arts, as a young man, Grandmaster Joe Greenstein once was shot between the eyes with a .38 - .40 caliber revolver by a man jealous of his wife. He walked out of the hospital the same day. Joe became very interested in the powers of the mind, since he survived this shot at the 'third eye' used in Buddhist meditation.

Martial meditation can bring the body's internal energy to a high level, so a basic background in meditation is presented along with specific martial consciousness concepts.

Internal energy physics, analogies and metaphors present a wide range of viewpoints to familiarize one to Qi (Chi) in the beginning chapter Physics of Internals. This provides a multimedia exposure to those beginning studies in internal energy.

SHAOLIN
SCHOOL LINEAGE

When the Ching soldier burned the Shaolin Temple in the 1700s, School Lineage from The Burning of Honan Shaolin Temple 1732 AD by Ching soldiers, thirteen monks escaped, with five traveling south and eight traveling north. Monk Chi Yuan went to Shantung province:

Monk Chi Yuan, Feng Shao Ch'en, Hsu Wei San, Yim Po, Yim Chi Wen, Kuo Yu Chang, Yim Shan Wu, Wong Jack Man

HSING-I
SCHOOL LINEAGE

- **Ji Long Feng**
- **Cao Ji Wu**
- **Dai Ling Bang**
- **Li Nen Ran**
- **Kuo Yun Shen & Li Kui Yuan**
- **Sun Lu Tang**
- **Kuo Yu Chang**
- **Yim Shan Wu**
- **Wong Jack Man**

There are three basic branches of Hsing-i: Honan, Hupei and Shanxi. Sun Lu Tang learned Hupei (Hubei) branch then added his theories and modified the sets so it is like a sub-branch of Hupei. The elements are fundamentally the same.

Kuo Yu Chang
(Gu Ruzhang)

Kuo Yu Chang's kung fu was at a very high level. Because his iron palm was so good, he was nicknamed "Iron Palm Kuo Yu Chang". His hands were soft as cotton which was not unusual. When he used his hands, it smashed rocks into many pieces and could bend raw iron. Many Kwangchou people have seen him take ten tiles, one on top of another, strike the first tile, and the tiles between the top and the bottom tiles broke into pieces, but both the top and bottom tiles remained intact.

First Demonstration of Kuo Yu Chang in 1925, Kuo Yu Chang's iron palm abilities were witnessed by a certain Hwang Hsien Sheng. To summarize the story, a Russian circus had posted an open challenge to anyone who would dare take three kicks from one of their horses. Anyone who survived would receive $1000 in gold, a huge sum of money at that time. Kuo Yu Chang accepted the challenge under one condition; instead of money, Kuo asked to strike the horse with one slap of his palm. The Russian owners of the circus accepted his conditions. In front of a huge crowd, the horse raised his hind leg and kicked Kuo in the chest. The crowd was silent in disbelief. Kuo then gathered his strength and when the horse kicked Kuo a second time, the crowd roared. When the horse kicked Kuo a third time, the crowd gave Kuo a huge ovation. Kuo then rested for more than half an hour. When he returned, he struck the horse in the rear, and the horse fell dead. Again, the crowd cheered at this incredible feat.

The famed Eagle Claw master, Lau Fat Meng, witnessed the postmortem on the horse. He observed that there was no external wound on the horse but that inside there was a large bruise on the horse's back and some of the horse's internal organs had been badly damaged.

In 1931, a strong man from Russia came to Kwangchou at west Mellon Garden (now near the People's Southern Road Kwangchou's Daily News Neighborhood), to exhibit strength feats. Anyone that could withstand a kick from the horse, would receive $200.00. The strong man observed that Kuo Yu Chang appeared to be an uncommon man and worried.

He demanded Kuo Yu Chang have an examination by a medical doctor to insure that he was a normal human. He got near the horse and using his palm lightly slapped it on the back. Immediately the horse stopped moving. On the second day, the horse did not eat and died. The doctor autopsied the horse and found severe internal injuries. The Russian quietly packed and left. This event of the 1930's is still much talked about among the old Kwangchou people today.

GRANDMASTER JOSEPH GREENSTEIN
(The Mighty Atom)
Wide Circle Kung Fu
Iron Palm, Iron Shirt (Golden Bell & Cotton Belly)

Greenstein became one of the 20th century's leading strongmen, standing only 5'4" and weighing 140 pounds. Demonstrations of strength included:

Using his hands to drive 20 penny nails through a 2 1/2 inch board;
supporting a 14-man band on his chest while lying on a bed of nails;
using his braided hair, pulling 32 tons of trucks coupled together;
breaking three chains by chest expansion;
bending 1/2 inch steel bars;
biting through a tempered railroad spike, using only his teeth.

During World War II, the "Mighty Atom" volunteered to help to recruit men for New York City's diminishing police force. He toured the city for two years giving demonstrations of jujitsu, judo, etc., to interest men in joining the civilian Police Force. He was highly commended by the Mayor and other officials of New York City.

Back in 1936, when six giant longshoremen became disorderly and tried to interfere with one of his associates who was lecturing. "The Atom," after a dramatic fight, put all six men in the hospital. Many of the New York papers carried a front page story entitled "Little Giant Knocks Out Six" The story read, "He weighs but 148 pounds, and is only 5'4 1/2" tall. No wonder writers have termed The Mighty Atom as "The World's Biggest Little Man."

He used Asian techniques of concentration, Jewish mystical writings, and a natural vegetarian diet.

Resisting the pull of a plane with his hair at the Buffalo Airport and was recorded in the Buffalo Evening Times on September 29, 1928.

He was featured several times in Ripley's Believe It Or Not and in the 1976 Guinness Book of World Records. In 1977, in his eighties, he received a standing ovation at his Martial Arts Show in Madison Square Gardens.

GRANDMASTER WONG JACK MAN
(Wong Chia Man)
By Robert Louie

'Wong Chia Man was born in Tai Shan (Toyshan), Kwangtung Province, China in 1941. He started learning Northern Shaolin Chuan in Central Park Canton, China, at the age of 8 years old from Yim Shan Wu who was Kuo Yu Chang's top disciple. In 1957, Wong Chia Man continued his lessons with Great Grandmaster Yim in Hong Kong. His talents were recognized by his Sifu and was one of the few selected to learn Northern Shaolin Lo Han from Great Grandmaster Ma Ching Fung, who learned from Kuo Yu Chang and Sun Yu Fung, King of Sabers. After years of learning both styles simultaneously, he received another letter of introduction (as the first letter of introduction was from Great Grandmaster Yim to Great Grandmaster Ma) from Great Grandmaster Ma to Great Grandmaster Yip Yee Ting of Mi Tsung Lo Han Chuan. After fifteen years of day and night study, Wong Sifu was highly trained and was the first person to complete the program studies in the Northern Shaolin Arts since World War II.

In the early 1960's Wong Sifu came to the United States of America in hopes of opening America's first Jing Mo Association. During the early years in America, he was practicing in the G & U Association where he would demonstrate his skills that he learned in the old country. As one elderly witness in the association states, "I witness Wong Sifu break a two inch wooden board against the grain with one light slap of his open palm. This demonstration illustrated how incredible his intrinsic energy really is." After practicing a number of years at G & U Association, Wong Sifu opened the first Jing Mo Association in San Francisco in 1964.

Wong Sifu's curriculum was a combination blend of the Standard Jing Mo School sets, Northern Shaolin, Northern Shaolin Lo Han, Northern Shaolin Lui Ho for the external styles and Sun's Hsing I, and Yang's Tai Chi and Li's Wu tang Swords for the internal styles. In 1969, his school became the largest martial arts school with students numbering in the hundreds in the San Francisco Bay Area.'

Some former students of Wong Jack Man:
Grandmaster Paul Eng
Wing Lam
Robert Louie, Rick L. Wing, Arthur Chin, and Herb Leung
Brent Hamby
Joseph Crandal
Al Dacascos
Peter Ralston

Jing Mo

Long ago, Jing Mo was started in Shanghai, China in March 1909, and the credit is given to the My Jong master and Chinese hero Fawk Yuen Gap (Ho Yuan Chia in Mandarin), who unfortunately passed away soon after in October 1909 from an illness. Many schools using the Jing Mo name have proliferated across the entire world, some connected with the main organization in Shanghai, others not.

Note that the name 'Jing Mo' is the Cantonese rendering, and it might also be spelled 'Ching Mo'. If people were to give the school a mandarin name, then they might called it 'Jing Wu', or 'Ching Wu'. The spelling in the English language does not seem to be totally consistent, so we mention this just to dispel confusion.

Other renderings of the words 'Tai Yook Woey' in English might be gymnastic association, sports club, physical culture association, and the like.

The Jing Mo Athletic Association was first brought to San Francisco in the early 1960's by Grandmaster Wong Jack Man. The school was also called 'The Chinese Physical Culture Association'. Grandmaster Wong is widely known among martial artists all over the world.

From the early 1960's to 1978, Grandmaster Wong taught martial arts in San Francisco's Chinatown, his main gung-fu school located for many years at 880 Pacific Avenue. A large black sign with white Chinese calligraphy saying 'Jing Mo Tai Yook Woey' hung above the entrance. The characters were written from right to left in the old Chinese style. He instructed students in the arts of Hsing-I, Tai Chi, Northern Shaolin, and various other styles of northern martial arts.

Wong Jack Man and Bruce Lee's Private Match

"BRUCE LEE'S TOUGHEST FIGHT", by Michael Dorgan (from Official Karate, July 1980)

Considering the skill of the opponents and the complete absence of referees, rules, and safety equipment, it was one hell of a fight that took place that day in December. It may have been the most savagely elegant exhibition of unarmed combat of the century. Yet, at a time when top fighters tend to display their skills only in huge closed-circuited arenas, this battle was fought in virtual secrecy behind locked doors. And at a time when millions of dollars can ride on the outcome of a championship fight, these champions of another sort competed not for money, but for more personal and passionate reasons. The time was late winter, 1964; the setting was a small kung fu school in Oakland, California. Poised at the center of the room, with approximately 140 pounds packed tightly on his 5'7" frame, was the operator of the school, a 24-year old martial artist of Chinese ancestry but American birth who, within a few years, would skyrocket to international attention as a combination fighter/film star. A few years after that, at age 32, he would die under mysterious circumstances. His name, of course, was Bruce Lee. Also poised in the center of the room was another martial artist. Taller but lighter, with his 135 pounds stretched thinly over 5'10", this fighter was also 24 and also of Chinese descent. Born in Hong Kong and reared in the south of mainland China, he had only recently arrived in San Francisco's teeming Chinatown, just across the bay from Oakland. Though over the next 15 years he would become widely known in martial arts circles and would train some of America's top martial artists, he would retain a near disdain for publicity and the commercialization of his art, and consequently would remain unknown to the general public. His name: Wong Jack Man.

What happened after the fighters approached the center of the room has become a chapter of Chinatown's "wild history," that branch of Chinese history usually anchored in fact but always richly embellished by fantasy, a history that tells much about a time and place with little that's reliable about any particular incident. Exactly how the fight proceeded and just who won are still matters of controversy, and will likely remain so. But from the few available firsthand accounts and other evidence, it is possible to piece together a reasonably reliable picture that reveals two overriding truths. First, considering the skill of the opponents and the complete absence of referees, rules, and safety equipment, it was one hell of a fight that took place that day in December. And second, Bruce Lee, who was soon to rival Mao Tse Tung as the world's most famous Chinese personality, was dramatically affected by the fight, perhaps fatally so.

Due to the human desire to be known as an eye witness to a famous event, it is easier to obtain firsthand accounts of the fight from persons who were not there than from those who were. As to how many persons actually viewed the contest, even that is a point of dispute. Bruce Lee's wife Linda recalls a total of 13 persons, including herself. But the only person that she identifies other than her husband and his associate James Lee, who died of cancer shortly before her husband died, is Wong Jack Man. Wong, meanwhile, remembers only seven persons being present, including the three Lees. Of the three persons other than the Lees and himself, only one, a tai chi teacher named William Chen (not to be confused with the William Chi Cheng Chen who teaches the art in New York), could be located. Chen recalls about 15 persons being present but can identify none other than Wong and the Lees. So except for a skimpy reference to the fight by Bruce Lee himself in a magazine interview, we are left with only three firsthand accounts of the battle. They are accounts which vary widely.

Linda Lee, in her book Bruce Lee: The Man Only I Knew, initially dismisses the fight as follows: "The two came out, bowed formally and then began to fight. Wong adopted a classic stance whereas Bruce, who at the time was still using his Wing Chun style, produced a series of straight punches. "Within a minute, Wong's men were trying to stop the fight as Bruce began to warm to his task. James Lee warned them to let the fight continue. A minute later, with Bruce continuing the attack in earnest, Wong began to backpedal as fast as he could. For an instant, indeed, the scrap threatened to degenerate into a farce as Wong actually turned and ran.

But Bruce pounced on him like a springing leopard and brought him to the floor where he began pounding him into a state of demoralization.

"Is that enough?" shouted Bruce. "That's enough!" pleaded Wong in desperation. So the entire matter was just another quick triumph for the man who frequently boasted he could whip any man in the world. Or was it? Later in her book, Linda Lee hints that the fight may have amounted to more than the brief moment of violent diversion she had earlier described. "Bruce's whole life was an evolving process - and this was never seen to greater effect than in his work with the martial arts," she begins. "The clash with Wong Jack Man metamorphosed his own personal expression of kung fu. Until this battle, he had largely been content to improvise and expand on his original Wing Chun style, but then he suddenly realized that although he had won comparatively easily, his performance had been neither crisp of efficient. The fight, he realized, ought to have ended within a few seconds of him striking the first blows - instead of which it had dragged on for three minutes. In addition, at the end, Bruce had felt unusually winded which proved to him he was far from perfect condition. So he began to dissect the fight, analyzing where he had gone wrong and seeking to find ways where he could have improved his performance. It did not take him long to realize that the basis of his fighting art, the Wing Chun style, was insufficient. It laid too much stress on hand techniques, had very few kicking techniques and was, essentially, partial."

Still later in the book, Linda Lee adds: "The Wong Jack Man fight also caused Bruce to intensify his training methods. From that date, he began to seek out more and more sophisticated and exhaustive training methods. I shall try to explain these in greater detail later, but in general the new forms of training meant that Bruce was always doing something, always training some part of his body or keeping it in condition."

Whether Bruce Lee's intensified training was to his benefit or to his destruction is a matter to be discussed later. For now, merely let it be observed that the allegedly insignificant "scrap" described early by Linda Lee has now been identified by her as cause for her husband to intensify his training and serves as the pivotal reason for his abandoning the fighting style he had practiced religiously for more than 10 years.

That the fight with Wong was the reason Lee quit, and then later repudiated the Wing Chun style, was confirmed by Lee himself in an interview with Black Belt. "I'd gotten into a fight in San Francisco (a reference, no doubt, to the Bay Area rather than the city) with a Kung-Fu cat, and after a brief encounter the son-of-a-bitch started to run. I chased him and, like a fool, kept punching him behind his head and back. Soon my fists began to swell from hitting his hard head. Right then I realized Wing Chun was not too practical and began to alter my way of fighting."

For those who have difficulty believing that a quick if clumsy victory over a worthy opponent was sufficient reason for Lee to abandon a fighting style that had seen him through dozens of vicious street fights as a youth in Hong Kong, where his family had moved shortly after his birth in San Francisco, a more substantial reason for Lee to change styles can be found in the account of the fight given by Wong Jack Man.

According to Wong, the battle began with him bowing and offering his hand to Lee in the traditional manner of opening a match. Lee, he say, responded by pretending to extend a friendly hand only to suddenly transform the hand into a four-pronged spear aimed at Wong's eyes.

"That opening move," says Wong, "set the tone for Lee's fight." Wing Chun has but three sets, the solo exercises which contain the full body of technique of any style, and one of those sets is devoted to deadly jabbing and gouging attacks directed primarily at the eyes and throat. "It was those techniques," say Wong, "which Lee used most."

There were flurries of straight punches and repeated kicks at his groin, adds Wong, but mostly, relentlessly, there were those darting deadly finger tips trying to poke out his eyes or puncture his throat. And what he say he anticipated as serious but sportsmanly comparison of skill suddenly became an exercise in defending his life.

Wong says that before the fight began Lee remarked, in reference to a mutual acquaintance who had helped instigate the match, "You've been killed by your friend." Shortly after the bout commenced, he adds, he realized Lee's words had been said in earnest.

"He really wanted to kill me," says Wong. In contrast to Lee's three Wing Chun sets, Wong, as the grand master of the Northern Shaolin style, knew dozens. But most of what he used against Lee, says Wong, was defensive. Wong says he parried Lee's kicks with his legs while using his hand and arms to protect his head and torso, only occasionally delivering a stinging blow to Lee's head or body. He fought defensively, explains Wong, in part because of Lee's relentless aggressive strategy, and in part because he feared the consequences of responding in kind to Lee's attempt to kill him. In pre-Revolutionary China, fights to the finish were often allowed by law, but Wong knew that in modern-day America, a crippling or killing blow, while winning a victory, might also win him a jail sentence.

That, says Wong, is why he failed to deliver a devastating right-hand blow on any of the three occasions he had Lee's head locked under his left arm. Instead, he says, he released his opponent each time, only to have an even more enraged Bruce Lee press on with his furious attack. "He would never say he lost until you killed him," says Wong. And despite his concern with the legal consequences, Wong says that killing Lee is something he began to consider. "I remember thinking, 'If he injures me, if he really hurts me, I'll have to kill him."

But according to Wong, before that need arose, the fight had ended, due more to what Linda Lee described as Lee's "unusually winded" condition than to a decisive blow by either opponent. "It had lasted," says Wong, "at least 20 minutes, maybe 25."

Though William Chen's recollections of the fight are more vague than the other two accounts, they are more in alignment with Wong's than Lee's. On the question of duration, for example, Chen, like Wong, remembers the fight continuing for "20 or 25 minutes." Also, he cannot recall either man being knocked down. "Certainly," he says, "Wong was not brought to the floor and pounded into a 'state of demoralization.'"

Regarding Wong's claim that three times he had Lee's head locked under his arm, Chen says he can neither confirm or deny it. He remembers the fighters joining on several occasions, but he could not see very clearly what was happening at those moments.

Chen describes the outcome of the battle as "a tie." He adds, however, that whereas an enraged Bruce Lee had charged Wong "like a mad bull," obviously intent upon doing him serious injury. Wong had displayed extraordinary restraint by never employing what were perhaps his most dangerous weapons - his devastating kicks.

A principal difference between northern and southern Chinese fighting styles is that the northern styles give much more emphasis to kicking, and Northern Shaolin had armed Wong with kicks of blinding speeds and crushing power. But before the fight, recalls Chen, "Sifu Wong said he would not use his kicks; he thought they were too dangerous."
And despite the dangerous developments that followed that pledge, Chen adds that Wong "kept his word." Though Chen's recollections exhaust the firsthand accounts, there are further fragments of evidence to indicate how the fight ended.

Ming Lum, who was then a San Francisco martial arts promoter, says he did not attend the fight because he was a friend of both Lee and Wong, and feared that a battle between them would end in serious injury, maybe even death. "Who," he asks, "would have stopped them?" But Lum did see Wong the very next day at the Jackson Cafe, where the young grand master earned his living as a waiter (he had, in fact, worked a full shift at the busy Chinatown restaurant the previous day before fighting Lee). And Lum says the only evidence he saw of the fight was a scratch above one eye, a scratch Wong says was inflicted when Lee went for his eyes as he extended his arm for the opening handshake.

"Some people say Bruce Lee beat up Jack Man bad," note Lum. "But if he had, the man would not have been to work the next day." By Lum's assessment, the fact that neither man suffered serious injury in a no-holds-barred battle indicates that both were "very, very good." Both men were no doubt, very, very, good. But Wong, after the fight, felt compelled to assert, boldly and publicly, that he was the better of the two. He did so, he says, only because Lee violated their agreement to not discuss the fight.

According to Wong, immediately following the match Lee had asked that neither man discuss it. Discussion would lead to more argument over who had won, a matter which could never be resolved as there had been no judges. Wong said he agreed.

But within a couple of weeks, he says, Lee violated the agreement by claiming in an interview that he had defeated an unnamed challenger. Though Lee had not identified Wong as the loser, Wong says it was obvious to all of Chinatown that Lee was speaking of Wong. It had already become common knowledge within the Chinese community that the two had fought. In response to Lee's interview, Wong wrote a detailed description of the fight which concluded with an open invitation to Lee to meet him for a public bout if Lee was not satisfied with Wong's account. **Wong's version of the fight, along with the challenge, was run as the top story on the front page of San Francisco's Chinese language Chinese Pacific Weekly**. But Bruce Lee, despite his reputation for responding with fists of fury to the slightest provocation, remained silent.

Now death has rendered the man forever silent. And the question of whether Wong presented Lee, who is considered by many to have been the world's top martial artist, with the only defeat of his adult life will remain, among those concerned about such matters, forever a controversial one. Even those Bruce Lee fans who accepts the evidence as supportive of Wong's account of the fight may argue that the outcome would have been different had the two battled a few years after Lee had developed his own style, Jeet Kune Do. But while it is true that Jeet Kune Do provided Lee with a wider range of weapons, particularly kicks, it is also true that Wong continued to grow as a martial artist after the fight. Only after that battle, says Wong, did he develop tremendous chi powers from the practice of Tai Chi, Hsing I, and Pakua.

Martial art styles can be divided roughly into two categories: external and internal. External styles, which are also called "hard" styles and which include such American favorites as Japanese karate and Korean taekwondo, rely primarily upon muscular strength, while internal or "soft" styles, such as Japanese Aikido and the three above-mentioned Chinese styles, cultivate a more mysterious energy called chi.

Although everybody has chi, few people have much of it, and fewer still know how to express it. But according to the Chinese, this precious elixir can be cultivated and controlled through the exercises of the internal martial arts styles.

Specifically, they say chi can be brewed in the tan tien, a spot about an inch below the navel. Once the tan tien is filled, the chi supposedly spills out into other parts of the body, where it is stored in the marrow of the bones. It is said that as a martial artist develops chi energy, his bones become hard, his sinews tough, is muscles supple and relaxed, which allow the chi to circulate freely through the body.

Chi usually takes much longer to develop than muscular strength, but it is considered a much more formidable energy. In normal times it is said to serve as a source of extraordinary vitality and as a guardian against many diseases. And in battle, it is said to provide a person with awesome power and near invulnerability.

Though Wong had been trained in the internal styles while still in China, up until the time he fought Lee he had concentrated mainly on the refinement of his elegantly athletic Northern Shaolin, which, like Lee's Wing Chun, is an external style. Following the battle with Lee, Wong would train in the internal styles until he had developed such chi power that he can, according to Peter Ralston, a former student of Wong and the first non-Asian to win the Chinese Martial Arts World Championships in Taiwan, take a punch to any part of his body without injury or even discomfort. As for Wong's offensive capabilities, they have apparently never been tested.

Regarding the question of how much Lee grew as a martial artist after the fight, Wong is convinced that the benefits to Lee from his homemade style were more than offset by the damage it did him. Wong even goes so far as to speculate that Jeet Kune Do may have caused Lee's death.

Most martial arts masters agree that just as serious training in a proper method can greatly improve one's health, strenuous and prolonged training in an improper method can destroy health. Often the health damage is attributed to improper breathing practices, and often the damage is to the brain. Special use of the breath is acknowledged by every martial arts style as a key element to developing power, though different styles have different breathing methods. Proper methods can be simply categorized as those which develop power while building health, and improper methods as those which either fail to build power or build it but at the expense of one's health. Though many of the ways in which breathing methods affect health remain mysterious, the methods themselves - at least the proper methods - have been empirically refined over many generations.

Wong's Northern Shaolin, for example, can be traced back to the great Shaolin Temple of more than a thousand years ago, which is considered the source of Chinese martial arts. While the Wing Chun practiced by Lee until his fight with Wong also had a long period of development and refinement, the style he put together after the fight was a chop suey of many and varied ingredients.

That Jeet Kune Do lacked the cohesion and harmony of a style in the traditional sense was something acknowledged by Lee himself, who preferred to call it a "sophisticated form of street fighting" rather than a style. After abandoning Wing Chin, Lee developed a disdain for all traditional styles, which he considered restrictive and ineffective. He even went so far as to place outside his school a mock tombstone that read: "In memory of a once fluid man crammed and distorted by the classical mess." It is grimly ironic that it would be Lee would be in need of a tombstone long before the man, trained by and loyal to the "classical mess," who was almost certainly his most formidable opponent.

It cannot be proven, of course, that Lee's fatal edema of the brain was caused by Jeet Kune Do, just as it could not be proven his death was brought on by any of the other rumored causes ranging from illicit drugs to excessive sex to blows on the head. Wong thinks, to serve as a caution to those who believe they can, by themselves, develop the knowledge it has taken others many generations of cumulative effort to acquire.

Perhaps it is because he gives so much credit to those who came before him that Wong's voice is absent of boast when he says his art was superior to Lee's. But while to him that is a matter of simple fact, Wong, aware that legends are larger than men, is not optimistic about ever being accepted as the winner of the fight. He says, however, that what people think regarding the outcome of the fight is less important to him than what they think provoked the battle in the first place.

In Linda Lee's account, which has been repeated in a number of Bruce Lee biographies, Wong is portrayed not only as a loser but also as a villian. According to Ms. Lee, Wong provoked the fight in an attempt to force her husband to stop teaching Kung Fu to Caucasians.

After sketching a brief history of Chinese martial arts up to the Boxer Rebellion, she writes: "Since then - and the attitude is understandable - Chinese, particularly in America, have been reluctant to disclose these secrets to Caucasians. It became an unwritten law that the art should be taught only to Chinese. Bruce considered such thinking completely outmoded and when it was argued that white men, if taught the secrets, would use the art to injure the Chinese, he pointed out that if a white man really wanted to injure a Chinese, there were plenty of other ways he could do it. "However, Bruce soon found that at first his views were not shared by members of the Chinese community in San Francisco, particularly those in martial arts' circles. Several months after he and James Lee had begun teaching, a kung fu expert called Wong Jack Man turned up at Bruce's kwoon (school) on Broadway. Wong had just recently arrived in San Francisco's Chinatown from Hong Kong and was seeking to establish himself at the time, all his pupils being strictly pure Chinese. Three other Chinese accompanied Wong Jack Man who handed Bruce an ornate scroll which appears to have been an ultimatum from the San Francisco martial arts community. Presumably, if Bruce lost the challenge, he was either to close down his Institute or stop teaching Caucasians."

So by Linda Lee's account, her husband had suddenly found himself in a position no less heroic than of having to defend, possibly to the death, the right to teach Caucasians the ancient Chinese fighting secrets. It is a notion that Wong finds ridiculous.

The reason he showed up at Lee's school that day, says Wong, is because a mutual acquaintance had hand-delivered a note from Lee inviting him to fight. The note was sent, say Wong, after he had requested a public bout with Lee after Lee had boasted during a demonstration at a Chinatown theater that he could beat any martial artist in San Francisco and had issued an open challenge to fight anyone who thought he could prove him wrong. As for those in attendance at the fight, Wong says he only knew of few of them, and those barely. Certainly, he says, no group had come as formal representative of the San Francisco martial arts community. Wong attributes both Lee's initial challenge and his response to the same emotion, to arrogance. "If I had it to do over," he says, " I wouldn't." But while admitting to youthful arrogance, Wong strongly contests Linda Lee's allegation that he was guilty of trying to stop Bruce Lee from teaching Caucasians.

It is true, say Wong, that most - but not all - of his students during his first years were teaching were Chinese. But that was true, he adds, only because few Americans outside of Chinese communities had even heard of kung fu. Americans who then knew anything at all of the martial arts most likely knew of Japanese judo or karate. They would not hear of kung fu until several years later, when it would be made famous by the dazzling choreography's of Bruce Lee.

Far from attempting to keep kung fu secret and exclusive, Wong observes that his was the first school in San Francisco's Chinatown to operate with open doors. That the other kung fu schools then in existence conducted classes behind locked doors was due more to the instructor's fears of being challenged, say Wong, than to a refusal to teach Caucasians. Once Caucasians became interested in kung fu, it would be Wong who would train some of the best of them, including Ralston and several other leading West Coast instructors. And all of these students of Wong who currently teaches at San Francisco's Fort Mason Center would be taught for a monthly fee amounting to a fraction of the hourly rate (in some cases $500) charged by the man who allegedly fought for the right to teach them.

COMMENTARY
Most JKD people think that Wing Chun is mainly about trapping when in fact trapping only makes up about 2 percent of the art and is only used if the opportunity creates itself. I can see no reason why JKD places non Wing Chun footwork with Wing Chun hands, something that defies the point of the Wing Chun elbow position and power generation in the first place.

Bruce Lee, declared Wing Chun impractical after this match. Bruce's own account has him chasing after Wong hitting the back of his head etc and becoming unusually winded. For a start, why was he chasing after Wong in that manner? It's odd to use the Wing Chun punches and methods in a way they were never meant to be used and then complain they didn't work.

Next, Bruce claimed the fight took three minutes. Three minutes of continuous aggressive fighting would take the wind out of most people. From Lee's own accounts of this fight, let alone Wong's, it is clear upon examination that he had a lot to learn and did not go about things in the right way, 'at the time of that fight'.

Bruce Lee was so impressed with Wong Jack Man's skills that he wrote to WJM's teacher and requested lessons. GM Ma Kim Fung turned him away, But Bruce Lee found and convinced Shui Hon Sang, who was an older classmate of GM Ma. GM Shui taught BL at least two sets, Kung Lick Chuan and Jie Chuan (Jeet Kuan).

There is a 8mm film of Bruce Lee doing Bei Shaolin #5 or attempting to perform BSL#5. He paid someone to film Wong Jack Man who was demonstrating BSL#5 and then BL learned from that film. Bruce Lee then had himself filmed doing the same set but from what I understand the quality was obviously not the same.

If Bruce Lee won the fight as he claimed, then why did he adapt the fighting methods of the loser? Ever other martial artist studies the methods of the winner.

MARTIAL BACKGROUND

1971-75 studied the Wide Circle of Kung Fu School in New York City and Berkeley, California. This is a primarily Northern Shaolin based style also studied Cotton Belly, Golden Bell (Iron Shirt) and Internal Iron Palm, under Grandmaster Joseph Greenstein, headquartered in New York.

From 1971-74 Mo Duk Kwan Tae Kwon Do, under Master Kenny Yuen of Oakland California (former partner of Byong Yu).

1973-4 Hapkido with Master Minh, University of California Berkeley, California.

1971-74; Aikido with Jeff Wilbur, Ho Chi Minh Gymnasium, Berkeley.

1974-79, Nippon Kenko Juko Association of Grandmaster Okano, learning Shotokan from Mr.Tanaka, and Lou Correa, and Goju under Masa, Koko and Hiro; 1976 Aido Samurai Sword under Master Samurai Takahashi; Samurai Dojo, Oakland, California.

1974-76 studied Yang style Tai Chi and Ba Gua at the Chinese Cultural Center on University Avenue, in Berkeley.

1982-85 Ba Gua and Hsing-i under Mr. ST Ying, "The Old Man" at the Chinese Baptist Church in Berkeley.

From 1980-87 in the San Francisco/ Bay Area of California, under Grandmaster Wong Jack Man of San Francisco Jing Mo; studying Hsing-i, Praying Mantis, Tai Chi, Lui Ho, Lohan, push hands and Northern Shaolin.

Sifu Greg Hayes has taught Martial Arts at the Yoga Den in Juneau (now Rainforest Yoga), from 1991-1998; Juneau Public School's Community Schools, from 1991-2005; the Free University of Berkeley, California, from 1970-1972 and has been giving private lessons in Juneau, since 1995.

OBJECTIVE MARTIAL TESTS

How do you know that the forms and drills you are practicing, are martially effective?

Breaking; Internal or External?

Even an external breaking punch can damage. One trained in this will have breaking material fracture like a stone hitting glass, circular fractal symmetry.

Externally generated hard strikes are not preferred, although they have a valid limited use:
  great for crippling wrists and elbow in arm strikes;
  knocking out high kicks with ankle and knee attacks and
  for shattering noses.

One classic test for external breaking quickness, is for a partner to lightly hold a 2 inch breaking board at the top suspended by the index finger and the thumb, then you break it. If you are just strong or fast, the board will move and not break.

Many in martial arts; equate soft with non-breaking methods; and some say that to break one must be external. Although this is not false; it is oversimplified, since internally hard training methods are not taught in the West commercially. This superficial understanding only signifies popular trends.

Some good targets for external breaks, are body areas that shatter easily, and damage is severe, even when it destroys a small surface area. Such targets are the nose, joints, temple and ear areas. The test for a focused external break is for it to radiate evenly from the center of the impact, much like a rock hitting a glass plate.

An **objective** test to see if your breaks are using internal power; is to break boards or tiles, and examine the cleavage of the break.

An externally manifested break's pattern will be angular, irregular and jagged.

An internally generated break pattern is a symmetric wave; through the X or Y axis (horizontally or vertically), the finer particled the material, the shorter the wave length.

Is your Qi nothing more than a warm feeling or a graceful flow? How do you know if your internal sets are functional or nothing more than healthy ballet?

An objective test for an internal blow; is to have a soft material such as a four inch thick phone book placed over a volunteer's abdominal-intestinal area, who will feel the strike through the material. If the strike is mainly felt on the surface, it is still an external blow. If you are just moved back, it is no more than a shove. A flexible material is used to avoid the billiard ball effect. This is done from between two and four inches away, so as to avoid any potential energy that is just accumulated by momentum. Do not do this without a trained sifu. See the end of the book for details.

Without a test that is objective, it can be argued that success is imagined. Many in martial arts say that this Qi business is not powerful enough to fight with. One could always fight, but this has to be done with everyone that disagrees with you; not practical.

Some psychologists say that even some results in your own body, can be accomplished through self-hypnosis, such as feeling, or change in body temperature.

There are also unscrupulous teachers and schools, that will take your money and time, and let you practice the same dud for years. When it comes time to use it, it does not work.

Test your product **BEFORE** you need it, and make the necessary corrections to make it effective, even if that means training elsewhere.

PHYSICS of INTERNALS

Building large muscles, inhibits range of movement, over-emphasizes linear/tendon connections, is limited by bone structure, and will build the external at the price of the internal. A human, is a lot like a plant, the internal organs being like the root, and the limbs like the stem and leaves. A person is born, with only so much internal organs to support their life. When one develops more of the limbs, they are like a root bound plant, in a pot too small. Just look at the life span of weight lifters, or body builders. For the most part, it is the slender people that live to be over 80.

When one develops their large muscle groups, they use their tendons, much like a cable, which is linear. The way to develop maximum force, is to use the whole body, in a FLOWING motion, much like a whip, or wave action. Muscle based bones, get in the way of this, as they do not bend, and inhibit the whipping action.

There are some Shaolin schools, such as Hung Gar, that are primarily external, and do rely on some training using weights. Northern Shaolin, which is more internal, does not use weights as much nor in the same manner. Most of the best Kung Fu, Ba Gua and Tai Chi teachers, prohibit weight training, since most using weights emphasize a different lifting method.

One can do power lifting, to open channels up, and then do the internal exercises, with increased flow of energies. It is good to be active, since this keeps everything flowing, and working together. This is different than focusing on weights, if one is sold on this, then why not just train with weights exclusively, and wrestle, so they can be an Ultimate Fighting gorilla. No one at this time, who promotes a lot of weight training; has taken any international fighting championships in China.

Talking about knife defenses, body builders and weight trainers; bleed like hoses, with even the smallest cut. Their energy flow is primarily blood based, ignoring the body's other channels/meridians.

The connective tissues such as ligaments, and the small muscles that keep one's joints in place, are much more important for the body to focus a wave, water-like and/or whip motion.

Heavy upper body development, will tend to make one top heavy, and overly Yang based. For internal martial striking strength, strengthen the arms but the legs more; for the root, centering power and the ability to FOCUS THE WHOLE BODY.

The standing exercises emphasis, is to open up the channels, and develop the root, not endurance for the muscle groups. This is what gives one the ability to use internal strength.

Most proponents of heavy weight training, do not even know what an Internal Punch is, let alone the ability to use one. For this, the muscles are not flexed on contact, although they are not limp either. Concentrating on large muscle development, will cause a rigidity in the muscles; that inhibits flow.

Try bending a hose with water running quickly through it. Explain that with myopic theories of large muscle machinations. There are those who would try to explain nuclear energy as chemical, rather than making the qualitative jump to atomic theory.

In the target area of the stomach/abdomen/intestines, an internal blow from a distance of 1 inch, will cause much more damage than a karate/boxing blow, at full distance. Explain that with mass/velocity theory. All martial power is not confined to breaking. Ever hear of hemorrhaging, or concussion?

To only understand force that is linear based, on the physics equations of Mass, Velocity, Inertia, and Velocity: is a very small part of martial power. Try explaining the Internal Iron Palm technique of breaking a brick in the middle of a stack of bricks, with external theories.

Non-Euclidean Geometry can explain where parallel lines meet, Euclidean cannot. In the same manner non-analytical meditative consciousness deals with the essences and universality of internals.

Even within the world of western physics, many new theories are being further developed around wave theory and the power of orbiting circles (geo-magnetics and guidance systems).

The internal was discovered and developed through Taoism and Buddhism not physics. It would be wiser to adapt physics to the realities of the internal, rather than try to force the round circles of Qi and wave theory, into the square headed, self-centered analytical logic; that is culturally arrogant and so narrow in its focus, that it can be compared to the blinders on a horse.

Analytical experts cannot produce the internal effect themselves, so their after the fact explanations of phenomena produced by someone else, is not based upon any of the skill required for participation and results.

Any moron can claim to be a Monday Night Quarterback expert, AFTER the weekend's football game has already been played.

For the muscle-heads out there;
Where are the gears on a rocket?
Where are the muscles in an explosion?
Where is the mass in an explosion-jet?
These are all wave based, not some cables with motors.

Wave physics; which has only been under development since the late 1960's, has produced successful theory models in many new areas.

WONDERBREAD HEAD

When one begins to learn a new skill, most learn something quicker when the new unknown is related to something that the student already knows. This is limited to concepts that are similar, so this training method is initially effective for a beginner's understanding.

In studying a new energy and way of moving, this only suffices to put one in the general ball park of what the new concept is. The words and examples being used; are structured relative the student's old world view. This is translating the knowledge in terms that only approximate the meaning of the skill, energy and/or essence.

An advanced technical skill requires its own terms and language, many unique to the discipline. Even identically spelled words have different meanings within the confines of medicine, law and computers.

Wonderbread is notorious for being over processed and refined. This process is recognized by most as loosing most of the nutrients in favor of a bread that looks nice and white, and is cheap. Wholewheat bread has more nutritive value, but there are those that do not like it, since it is dark, different, or harder to chew. Wonderbread is a good example of what is lost when something is, overly refined, processed or analyzed.

A novice in chess uses checkerboard mentality, to concentrate on taking pieces or checking the king. An advanced student; acquires entirely new concepts of access, different moving pieces, multiple move strategy, and territory. A good chess player will sacrifice the taking of the number of pieces to win the game in gambits.

In mathematics, one's learning of the area of a curve; is arithmetically explained by calculating of square blocks within the curve. A precise calculation involves calculus, a new theory of differential functions.

Traditional Chinese Internal Martial Arts is qualitatively different than external martial arts. Some students learning TCIMA, have attained an advanced level of a move, that is externally good, relative to external martial artist's criteria. For some things this can help in leaning a new move, if it is similar, and the different energy and focus are applied. For other moves this is a student's trained and hardened response, which must be overcome. Sometimes close is not good enough. For these reasons many will not teach advanced concepts of the internal to those trained in externals, since it takes them longer to learn than if they had no training at all. Old concepts sometimes have to be shattered.

One's martial skill can be viewed as stick or bar moving through new fields, consciousnesses and planes. One can quantatively add to the length of the 'knowledge bar' with related facts. When this bar moves through 'sea of knowledge', the bar does not stretch; it looses occupied territory in its rear, in order to occupy more territory in the front. If one does not let go of the old concepts, one cannot grab the new concepts.

When one translates a different skill into imprecise old concepts, they are stretching relative meanings; which has only limited results.

Most with backgrounds in the external; are taught to throw their shoulder into a punch. Boxers and karateka add to the power of the arm contracting, so this does help some. Some of the better boxers like Ali, throw their hips into the punch with the move of the shoulders. Most of this is limited to a torso twist. Some of the most experienced boxers, and advanced karateka, time the forward punch's torso twist, with the hip twist. Even fewer time this with the step.

When one learns a front karate punch, they withdraw the opposite arm, to counter the forward striking hand; adding some power. The external emphasizes upper arm strength, and shoulder bulk; so this movement of the opposite arm; appears to be in reverse motion, but it is not. The physics and power of this move are affected by: how the arms are attached to the body, how the torso is mounted on the body's frame, and gravity's affect of the stance and leg power.

HSING-I BASICS

In the beginning of the movement, the body remains soft so Qi can be led to the limbs. Hsing-i Jin is similar to rattan, soft and bending, yet hard when it strikes. The power is manifested like a cannonball exploding.

Learning Hsing-i:
in the beginning it will appear simple and easy,
when first trying the move it will appear complicated and difficult,
after mastering Hsing-i, it will become direct and simple easily executed.

HSING-I ELEMENTS

Metal corresponds to the lungs
Water corresponds to the kidneys
Wood corresponds to the liver
Fire corresponds to the heart
Earth corresponds to the spleen.

CREATING ELEMENTS
metal creates water
water creates wood
wood creates fire
fire creates earth
earth creates metal

When practicing 5 elements, it is best to practice in creating order.

COUNTERING ELEMENTS
metal counters wood
wood counters earth
earth counters water
water counters fire

When practicing defensive responses; it is best to reply with the element that counters.

In Metal (Pi) the rising and drilling rear hand starts as a rising wave, passes its energy to the front hand and continues like a falling ax, the rear hand slides along the axe handle (a point from the base of the front hand to the Lower Dan Tien).

In Water (Zuan) the front hand first goes from palm upward to down blocking, as one would overturn a cup of water then passed and collected by rear hand with an outward to inward twist rooted on or below the ground. The rear hand which becomes the right hand, strikes with a spurting energy springing upward.

In Wood (Beng), the front hand downward blocks much like Tai Chi Brush Knee, which pulls the rear striking hand which shoots out like an arrow.

In Fire (Pao), the front rising hand blocks upward as it pulls rear hand which strikes out like a canon shooting.

In Earth (Heng), the front hand moves outside to inside with a circular ridge hand palm down, passes the energy to the rear hand that is palm up; as both hands follow each other in a small circle near the Lower Dan Tien tearing that energy like cotton cloth, propelling rear striking hand in an inside-to-outside strike-block. Elbows should be tucked.

BASICS

Since you are exercising your internals; it is best not to stress them with a full stomach, bladder or intestine.

When you practice, keep the whole body balanced.

No part of the body can lose balance. If the balance is even a little off, that is called "focus" or "double-weight." Focus is the mind feeling, and double weight the physical feeling.

Be natural and letting your reflexes work. This is not simple. You must understand these two ideas deeply.

In the martial arts there are two kinds of movements that are continuous, unbroken and from one root.

The eyes look straight ahead, the limbs and body are relaxed.
The mouth is closed, the tongue touches the roof of the mouth.
The entire soles of the feet grip the ground.
The middle of the sole of the foot, roots beneath the ground.
The "bubbling springs point" or yongquan cavity, Kidney 1, located between the mounts of the big, and second toe, on the sole of the foot; is contracted inward.

The fingers are stretched and opened.

Relax the shoulders and empty the chest, press the head upward and straighten the back of the neck.

Exhale smoothly, delicately, even slow and long.

At the top of the circle, begin to exhale, relax the anus area (Gu Dao or Huyin Point)
at the bottom, begin to inhale, lift up the anus area.
.

The elbows push the palms and hands.

Six Harmonies:
the hands harmonize with the heart
the shoulders harmonize with the hips
the elbows harmonize with the knees
the heart harmonizes with the intent
the intent harmonizes with the Qi (Chi)
the Qi harmonizes with the power.

Hsing-i is very yang, so you will not only heat up, but the room you are in will heat up also. Do not drink much when doing Hsing-i, as it will upset this yang effect.

Hsing-i can build on itself, gaining energy momentum, intensity, and waking you up. Many that do other internal martial arts will start with Hsing-i, do to its energizing effects.

The cumulative effects of Hsing-I line practice will heat and speed you up, as well as give you a surge of power. Passed energy from staging moves becomes more apparent as it carries you away. Do up to 10 repetitions in at least two different directions. Do some Hsing-I lines and get carried away.

The general trend for movement is to stretch upward for distance and to contract as you drop your weight/center root, as you strike. Rise to go, fall; for a strike: undulating as a dragon.

The moves are combinations of successive unfoldings of the separate steps of staged accumulated momentum: many moves merging into one, as a wave. This propelled sequence is an energy focus that goes through individual moving, transcending the particular form and time.

This could easily be compared to a paper-folding that has already been constructed, and is being opened to its desired expanded physical form.

HSING-I ENERGY FUNDAMENTALS

Energy Centers
Upper Dan Tien (third eye) is like a fog.
Middle Dan Tien (solar plexus) is like a pond.
Lower Dan Tien (below navel) is like a ditch.

Hold the chest,
stretch the back,
relax and sink the shoulders,
drop the elbows,
close up the body and rise,
lengthen the body and lower.

In Hsing-i, the feeling between the hands is often compared to tearing cotton, especially pronounced in Earth.

Slightly clenching the teeth and lightly raising the head;
focuses the mind intent, different than in Tai Chi.

The feet gripping the ground directs the wave of the move.

The feet carry the move, then the move carries the body; as if there were bungi chords or a Slinky (physics toy coil) between the feet. The power and grounding of the strike is squeezed from the feet, much like the organist's pedal play of an organ's foot chords.

In the step forward, the heels successively launch the plumb of the body moving forward as if leaping across a ditch.

The initial blocking hand fills the void, carrying the striking hand, as a wave in the surf. Successive forward upward moves stretch and unfolds next move, then contracts as it lowers a strike.

The tone of the strike is shaped by the Lower Dan Tien, as a guitar's notes are from the guitar body of an acoustic guitar.

The forms advance or retreat, but are never fixed. The head is pushed upward slightly, whereas in Tai Chi it is slightly suspended.

Both hands are unsettled winding above the center.

With the foot steps, the true idea is to not fall into emptiness. Disperse the breath. The issuing is totally in the rear foot. Store up the intent. You need to protect the groin. If the beginning posture is good, then use 'Sweeping the Ground Wind'.

Rooted steps are the scissor handles of the scissor-stepping that are driving the martial motion through one's Lower Dan Tien (scissor's axis pivoting point), that focuses the strike forward (scissor's cutting tip).

In every movement, watch your Yi. When Yi generates the idea for movement, the Qi will be immediately led to the end section, starting the movement of the end section. The middle section follows and the root section urges the movement. This is not the same as Tai Chi, because the body in Hsing-i is more like rattan than water. Even though it is flexible, the body is hard so when the Yi is generated on the target, the tip can move first, and the power is pushed from the body and the root section.

Stomp while advancing; as a one would off a trampoline to launch a strike.

SAN TI SHI STANCE (Metal)

Right rear leg is bent, toes pointed outward from the body, root goes from below the heel down 3-6 feet; bearing 60% -75% of body weight.

Left leg is in front, toes pointed forward, at right angle to rear foot, shoulder width away from the rear right leg.

Left arm is extended forward at about shoulder level, elbow lower than the hand. Left is ridge hand held vertically up, palm facing inward, thumb side inward. Lower Dan Tien flows Qi directly to hand heel.

Right arm is held forward, with the rear elbow near abdominal area, right hand at fully extended, palm down and slightly inward.
Lower Dan Tien flows Qi from right elbow through the arm which is held horizontally level, slightly tucked near the navel.
Right index finger points to left hand and right palm area flows Qi to left heel hand's base.

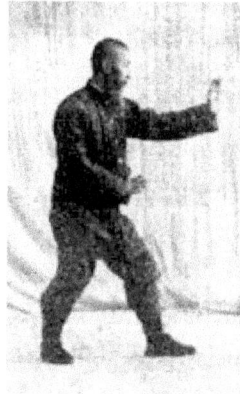

In the stance of San Ti Shi:

Root	Mid-section	Terminus
Hips	Knees	Feet

The shoulders push the elbows, the elbows push the hands, the waist pushes the hips, the hips push the knees, and the knees push the feet.

The knees should have the feeling as though they are closing inward and the heels should feel as if they are pushing outward.

Both knees bend inside with strength which does not manifest itself. The hips urge the knees.

Eyes looking to the tiger's mouth (acupuncture point Li-4), of forward hand, near where the index finger and thumb meet:
toes out at 60 degrees,
heart is as quiet as still water,
while the crown of the head gently presses upward,
the bai hui point at the crown part of the head,
has the feeling of being sucked inward;
chin gently tucked in,
the insides must be lifted,
when the feet kick, the whole body must be empty,
energy sinks to the Lower Dan Tien.

TERMS

Hsing-i, Hsing Yi, and Xing Yi are all the same, just spelling of different time periods

"Sink the waist", the coccyx must be relaxed and slightly uplifted, the yang will ascend toward heaven. This regulates the Du meridian

"Pressing the shoulders" is like practicing the steps, urge the rear as if erecting the waist, round the crotch to support the hips, lift the chest as if back bending.

"Shoulders", usually refers to the power of the "shoulder well point", sink down to the Yong Quan (k-1). When using the power of the shoulder well point, soften the intent and relax, there will be no obstruction. When relaxing the shoulders they feel as if they are being pulled back.

"Urging the rear" refers to squeezing the buttocks together as much as possible. The crotch feels as if it is pressing across both inwardly and outwardly with maximum effort.

"Lifting the chest" refers to lifting the chest as is resisting a force form the front. Relax the shoulders ass if youre putting forth strength. Both sides of the back bone press forcefully together, the energy originates from below the navel, from the internal organs revolving outward to the head and then returns.

"Hsing-i step method" is a four step process, initially in San-ti stance:
1) like a 'Slinky', the rear foot propels, the body forward as it steps forward, past the front leg as if it were to leap across a ditch;
2) as the rear leg passes the body's plumb center, it becomes the new front leg and one sinks into a lengthened stance (bow), into the new rear leg;
3) the rear leg follows the front leg's forward momentum in a bungi chord type connection: slightly shortening the stance, (San-ti): one sinks as the rear leg drives the flow of the front leg and the knee/Lower Dan Tien/elbow/hand strike;
4) the front leg goes with forward force changing to mid-length San Ti, front foot pedals the direction and focus of the hand strike, and sometimes front leg moves forward a little, as one sinks into the shortest stance.

HSING-I CONCEPTS

Some say upper body power comes from the returning hand; when the body is connected the back hand generates the power and moves like a wave through the torso and out the striking hand. The theory thinks that when only using the attacking arm, your power will be limited to the strength in the arm and your forward momentum.

This works fine for external karate. Internal Hsing-i does not have to be limited to the torso.

Internal Hsing-i has more emphasis in the internal concepts of Chi being generated and focused by the Lower Dan Tien and the Sacrum. Attacks do not rely on forward momentum, as I can externally puncture or break, within 2-4 inches, and internal strikes of 2 inches or less that can kill. Power is increased by the raising and lowering of the body, which is quicker and more stable than momentum based potential power, and relying on distance acceleration.

The returning hand can add limited power through basic Newtonian physics of an opposite reaction, through the torso, but this eliminates the connection to the Lower Dan Tien, the ground, and the center of the body's mass and Chi.

One embarking on learning a new method should not attempt to teach it, without 1,000-10,000 correct repetitions. Even this is not enough when one wants to make a qualitative leap, since a new method involves a total picture gained over multiple moves and forms, forged through years of practice, integration, testing and combat.

What is sometimes referred to as bioelectric energy, encompasses more than an understanding of Newtonian physics, and electricity. This is an entirely different energy, philosophy, and energy theory. One would do better to immerse themselves in the new concepts, imagery, and theory; rather than translate it.

A good teacher is critical to learning new perceptions, and new cognitive processes. These combine with the 'shared lived experience' and 'shared history' of the new Martial Art's language, focus, perceptions and mastery. Phenomenology and Buddhist meditation will aid this greatly.

Newtonian concepts of opposite reactions, are not necessarily a contributor to most moves, but some. Even within this narrow range, the effects in Traditional Chinese Internal Martial Arts apply to more than one plane. For most westerners, and sports buffs; this plane is further limited to the upper arm shoulder pivot, which is overly top heavy and Yang. Some of the other planes are Ying Yang opposites, and gravitational. Fluid dynamics comes closer to explaining internals than Newtonian.

In Classic Hsing-i, the opponent does not see the legs coming. One studying in Hsing-i for up to the first five years; tends to over emphasize the arm's relationship.

Eight Character Song (8 Triagrams)

Ding: push outwards, Kou: hook, Yuan: round, Min: quick, Bao: embrace, Chui: hang, Chu: curved, Ting: stretch out.

The back of the skull pushes upward, the palm pushes outward, and the back of the tongue pushes upward.

Hook: the shoulders, the backs of the hands and feet, and the teeth.

Round: the back, the front of the chest, and the hand's tiger mouth.

The mind, eyes and hands must be quick.

Embrace: the Dantien, mind/Qi, and the ribs.

The Qi, shoulders and elbows must hang. Some say that the shoulders move the elbows, but it is better to emphasize the embracing of the ribs by the elbows, which puts the hands closer to the lower Dantien, which moves the hands more than the skeletal elbow mechanics. More importantly the shoulders should be coordination with the hips.

Bow the arms, knees, and the wrists; like a half moon.

Stretch the neck, back and kneecaps.

Coordinate the shoulders to the hips, the elbows to the knees and the feet with the hands.

If the left shoulder is completely twisted, the right will naturally follow.

The arms are naturally bent, without bending being pronounced; naturally straight without being rigidly straight. If the arms are too straight, there will not be enough flow for strength, but if too curved they will not reach their target.

Keep the right hand by the ribs, the left by the chest, rub the rear hand, reach out with the front; between the hands, front and back, the proper use of strength is equal.

TRADITIONAL INTERNAL ENERGY WORKOUTS

STANDING POLE, EMBRACE THE M00N, ZHANG ZHUANG, TREE HUGGING, HOLDING THE BALL;

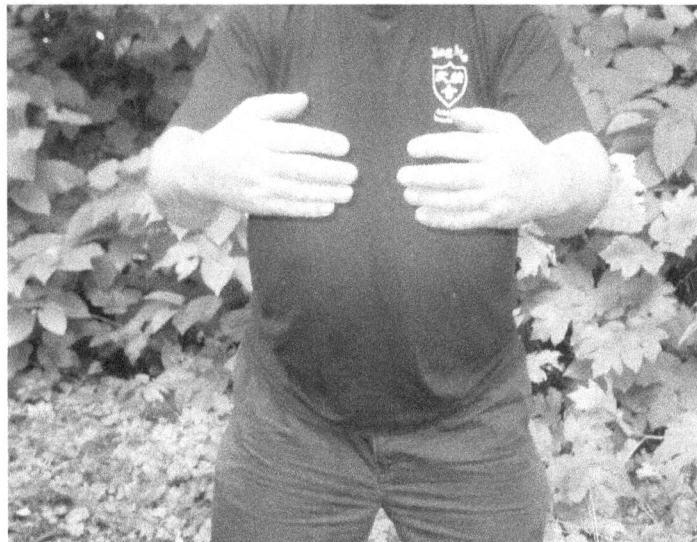

Hold the arms in a circle, elbows lower than hands, palms facing inward, thumb side on top with a gap between the opposing fingers of 1/4 - 4 inches apart, at a height:
  a) initially holding hands at solar plexus level,
  b) for more effort in the arms, one can raise the arm level up to a height of the chin, but this can cause overheating, and a loss of one's root and balance during prolonged standings; or
  c) gradually dropping the arms to any point between solar plexus level, to the Lower Dan Tien (a few inches below the navel).

Start with 10 minutes a day, then work up to being able to stand either:
a) 45 minutes with both legs parallel or
b) two sets of 30 minutes each, alternating leg forward, without dropping hands.

The intensity of the work is the foot and leg position and how far you sink. Through bringing the feet parallel, widening the stance and sinking lower you intensify it.

The extreme of full Riding Horse stance, is sinking until your thighs are parallel to the ground. The old traditional test was balancing a tea cup on your thigh.

Stand with both feet shoulder width apart and parallel. Legs should be straight but don't let the knee joint lock back. Hips and shoulders face square to the front, and the head is held upright.

Rock side to side until you feel your weight fall evenly from the crown of the head directly down the midline of your body, to extend between your legs beneath the ground from 3-6 feet. Next begin to rock slightly back and forward from heal to toes; find the place where the weight of the body is equally distributed between the heel and the ball of the foot.

Relax and extend the toes opening up and flattening the arch of the foot to create what we call an energy well. Now let the weight of the body fall down through this well in the bottom of each foot; dropping like a stone 3-6 feet below the ground. Arms relax by your side, relax your body but extend your spine and pull your head upwards. Breathe deeply through your nose using your stomach or diaphragm, not your chest.

Hollow the chest, relax the area between the eyes, and position the eyes to lightly gaze at the midpoint of the third eye. Next open the palms of the hands, palms facing inward, with fingers pointing to each other; thumb points to other thumb, index finger to other hand's index finger etc. Hands should not be overly flat, nor overly rounded; but slightly rounded. Draw your elbows out slightly to create a small space under the armpit. Do abdominal breathing through your nose, let the mind and the breath drop to your Lower Dan Tien (the space between the kidneys).

Draw in you chin so your head aligns with your spine. Relax the muscles of the mouth and jaw and lightly rest your tongue on the top of your mouth. Let your eyes be softly open but try not to look at anything specifically, take your mental attention away from the visual stimulation.

You should have the feeling of being hung by a thread attached to the top of your head like a puppet. You should feel your head floating effortlessly up and at the same time the weight of your body rooting through your feet 3-6 feet into the earth. Your energy below the ground; is the base of the pyramid, the head the point.

When you exhale, relax the anus area (Gu Dao or Huyin Point); as you inhale, lift up the anus area.

OUT & IN

Start in the horse stance, Standing Pole position described prior.

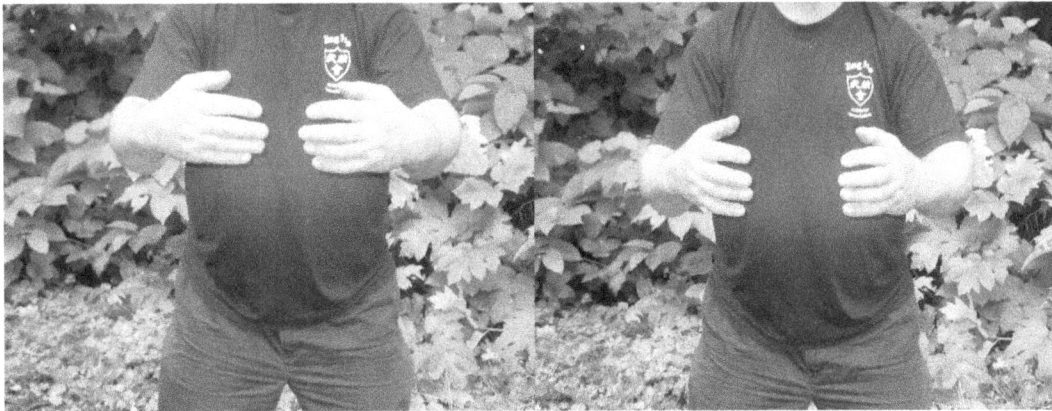

As you inhale, start to widen the gap between your knees from your feet pushing outward toward the outside of the feet; rising slightly.

Cradle your hips forward and upward

Increase the gap between the hands while expanding the abdominal area by the Lower Dan Tien, augmented by a slight expansion of the gap between the elbows and the rib cage. Back of the hand near the wrist, leads fingers and rest of the hand; as in Monkey, Crane and Praying Mantis.

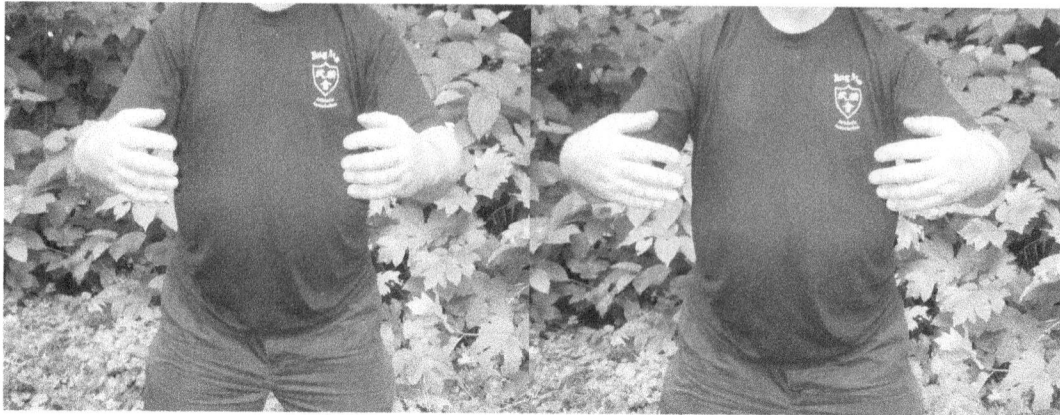

As you exhale; start to sink your root, while your feet's arches move inward and downward, driving the knees inward.

Cradle your hips backward and downward

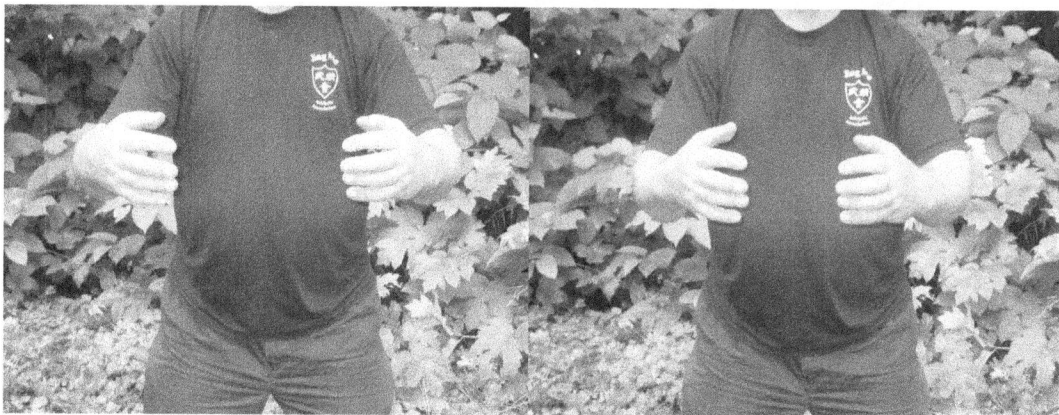

The contracting the abdominal area through the Lower Dan Tien; will urge the elbows to move slightly outward form the rib cage, which shortens the gap between the hands. Heel of the hand leads the rest of the hand inward. This returns you to the Standing Pole position.

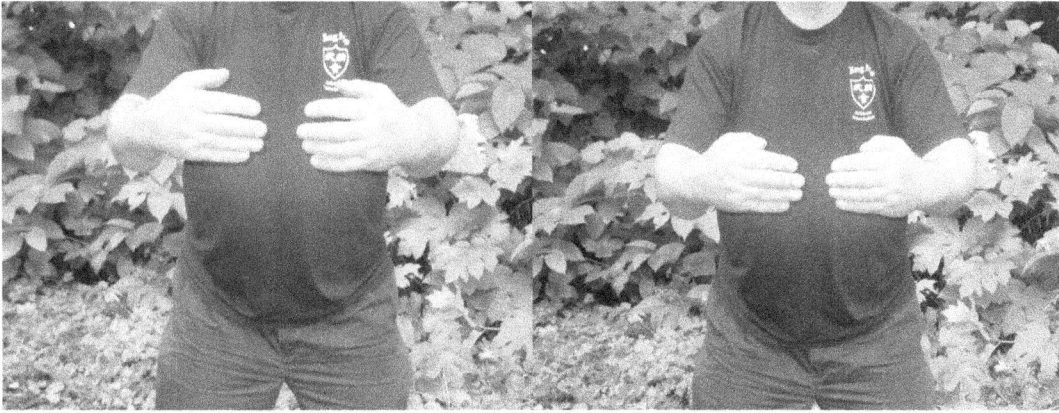

SHIFTING THE WATER

Side to Side

1) Start in the Standing Pole position in horse stance, weight evenly
   distributed between both legs, holding hands a little lower at
   abdominal height.

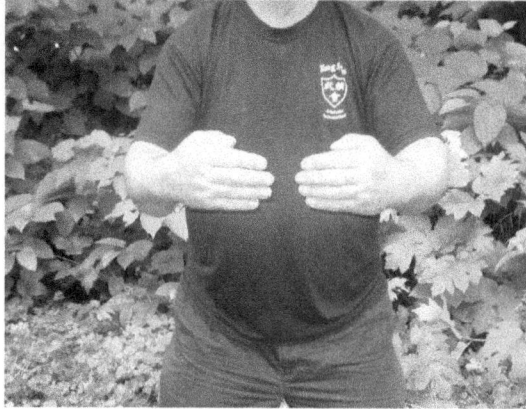

2) Slightly shift your stance from right to left by tilting the right foot,
   at the ankles; leftward, then bending the right knee inward,
   continuing this leftward movement with the hip.

3) Weight is shifted to the left side as the leftward movement crosses
   your midpoint, by bending the left knee.

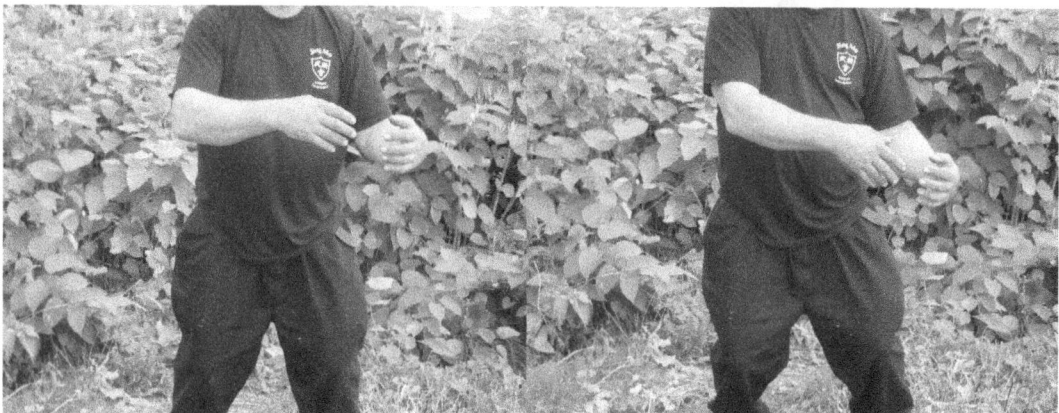

4) Chi (Qi) is poured like water, from the right hand's outstretched
   fingers, toward and into the left hand's palm as the body slightly
   tilts leftward.

5) Right leg is emptied of Chi, left leg is full.

6) The flow of Chi should transferred from side to side evenly from midpoint flowing through hand downward into the left leg and continuing this sinking down the feet to 3-6 feet beneath the ground.

7) Return to Standing Pole horse stance position with weight evenly distributed, by slightly shifting your stance from left to right by tilting the left foot, at the ankles; toward the center, slightly straightening the left knee then raising the left leg the right knee inward, continuing this rightward movement with the hip.

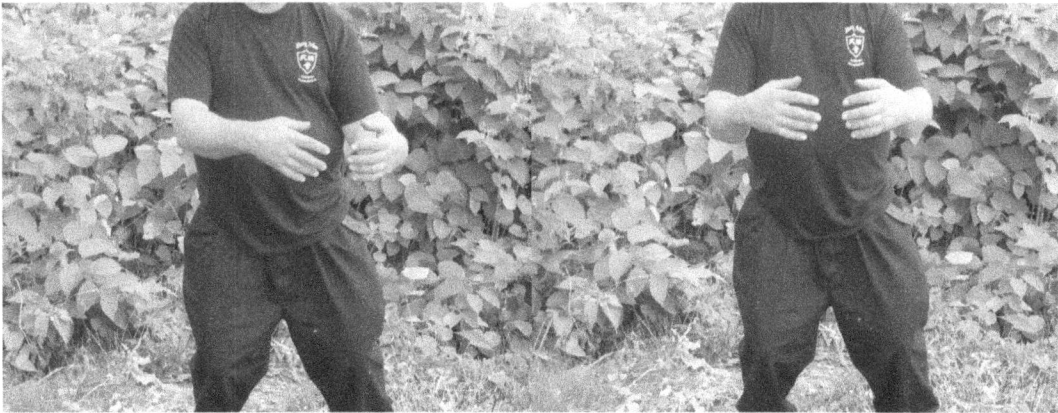

8) Shift from center to the right as described in 1) - 6) but with opposite sides.

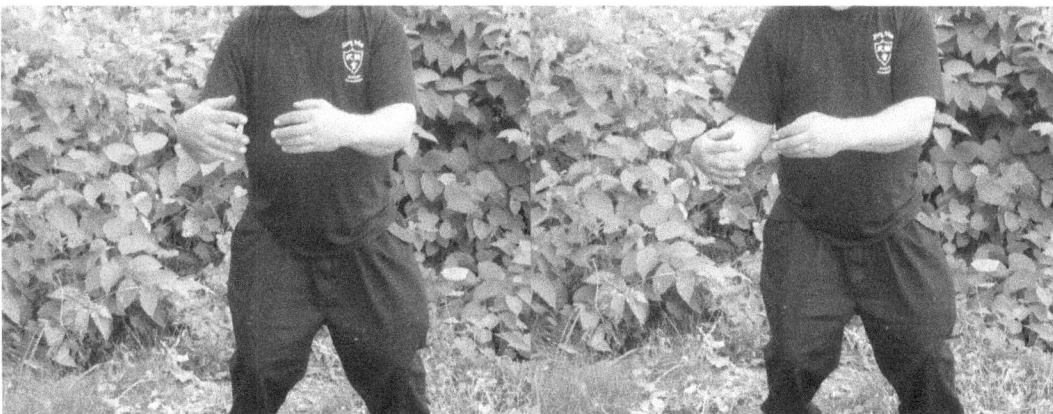

SHIFTING THE WATER

Back and Forth

1) Do Holding the Pole exercise in a San Ti Stance or a T Stance,
   with feet at right angles
   left foot forward bearing 1/3 of the weight, hands at abdominal height.

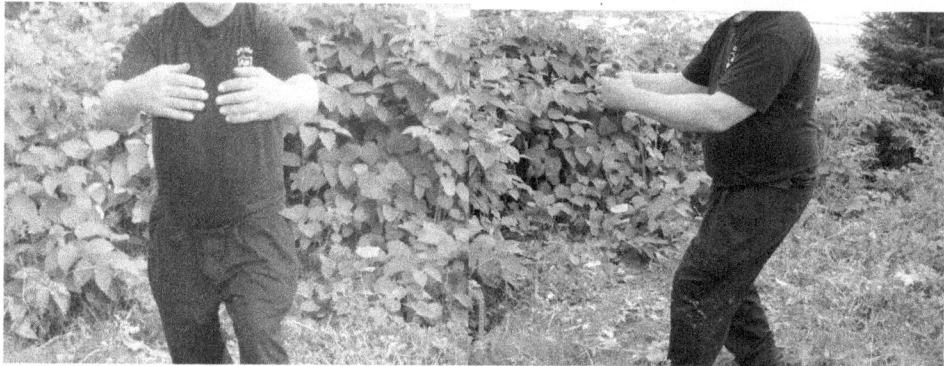

Next you will draw the paired arms downwards, and backwards with
the body as described in 2) - 4).

2) Bend the right rear leg at the knee; sinking into the ground beneath
   your right foot.

3) Shift more weight onto the right rear leg, through drawing the body
   backwards, by first angling the right ankle toward your ridge heel;
   shifting the weight of the left front foot onto its heel, with the toes
   pointing upward.

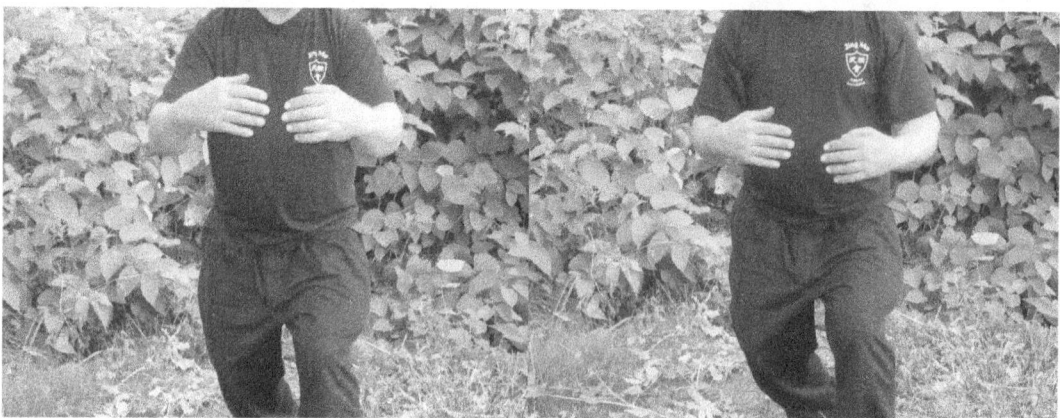

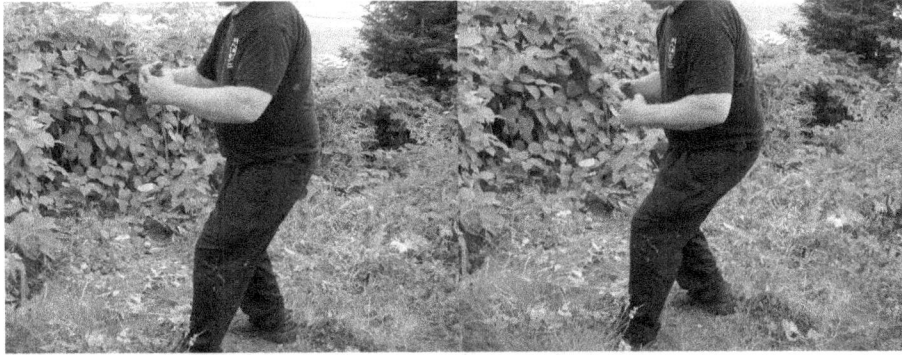

4) The rear right leg draws the Lower Dan Tien back and downward, the Lower Dan Tien draws the arms and hands back with it, the arm length shortening with the backwards draw. Right leg has all of the weight, and is full. Left leg has no weight on it and is empty. This completes the back and down movements.

5) Next there will be a push forward and upward.

6) Start the pushing up, by straightening the knee. You push forward by pushing from the right rear foot's ridge side, angling the foot forward, then the right knee forward; which moves the Lower Dan Tien forward. The Lower Dan Tien pushes the arm set forward as your arms are extended forward to their full length.

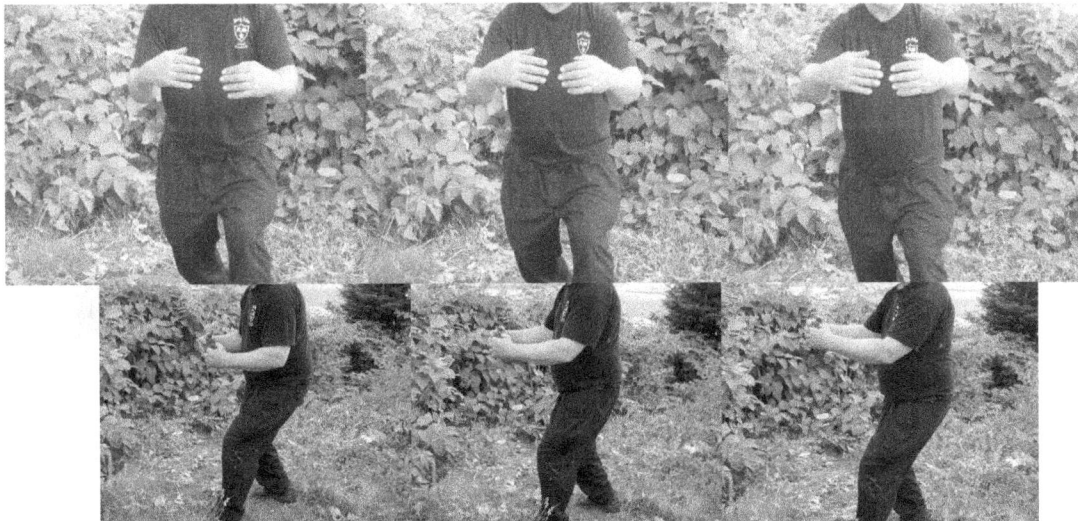

6) As the body is raised by the rear leg; 1/3 of the weight is shifted forward to the front foot, as the left front foot's toes comes down, flattening the foot.

7) Continue this upward and forward push, until you have returned to your original position in 1). Switch sides and repeat.

ROWING EXERCISE

Stand in a L version of the T-stance or Cat Stance: one foot in front pointed forward, the other (back) at right angels and bent, with 60-80 % of the weight on the back.

Your hands should be by your side, with the fingers relaxed, hands upheld slightly.

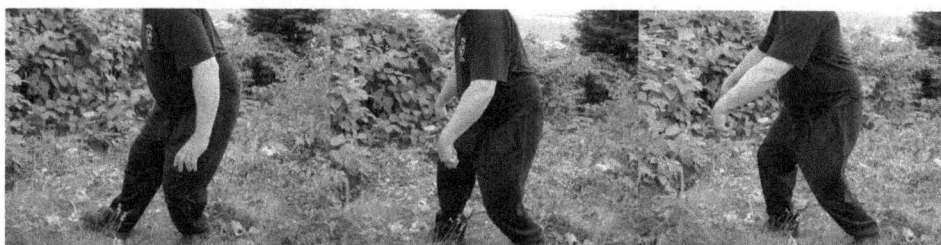

Push with the back leg and shifting your weight forward. This push should start at your root, below the ground and be guided by your ankles, to knees, to waist, where it is transferred, in a swinging motion, to ones arm/hands; into a hook hands (mantis or crane) position.

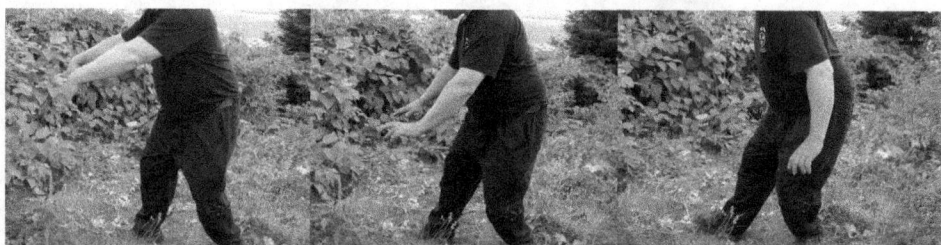

Now drop back toward the rear leg, shifting your weight back, as one would slosh water around in a jug; the water being your Qi, the jug being your body. Some call this a shifting of weight, but it is a better image to think of one leg becoming full (of Qi/weight), and the other being empty.

Perform the Rowing Exercise on a small boat or raft, you will see where your center, and momentum is.

Do the Rowing Exercise with each hand loosely holding gallon jugs of water, 2/3 full. Watch your momentum and flow. When you get better, try and have the sway, carry your next row/step.

Try doing the Rowing Exercise on ice, this will show the angle of your push, and your rooting, if ice is not available, oil, on a waxed floor, would substitute.

For the cross country skiers among you, use the rowing in your push off of the ski poles, for added power, and balance.

An old Shaolin exercise for this; is to walk up hill and/or on a narrow plank, carrying a 5 gallon bucket of water in each hand. Swaggering, and acting as if you were drunk (drunken style kung fu), while carrying the water; will show you where your Qi/Chi is.

UNBENDABLE ARM

Stand in a relaxed horse stance with one fully extended arm raised to the side. The arm should be slightly curved inward with fingers extended, palm up.

Flow energy from your Lower Dantien, through your arm and about 4 inches past your fingers.

This flow through your arm; is like the flow of water through a hose, except for the wetness.

A good example to try; is to attempt to bend a hose. While water is rushing through it, if it is a fire hose it will be impossible. Have a classmate attempt to bend the arm at the elbow. Your arm will be firm, but not the definition of tightly contracted muscles (bands separated and pumped).

Next check the arm by someone tapping the arm. It should not be flaccid or limp; yet it should sway slightly with the blow. If muscles are tense; it will not sway, only jerk. The firmness of the arm's meat; is similar to the touch of excellent muscle tone.

This muscle-meat is the conduit and capacitor of Qi.

PUSH INTO GROUND, PULLOUT FROM GROUND-ROOT

From a front Horse Stance:

Part 1,
Upheld hands gather heaven chi into Lower Dan Tien,
as one inhales and tucks the lower abdominal area,
gather a ball of energy in your palm.

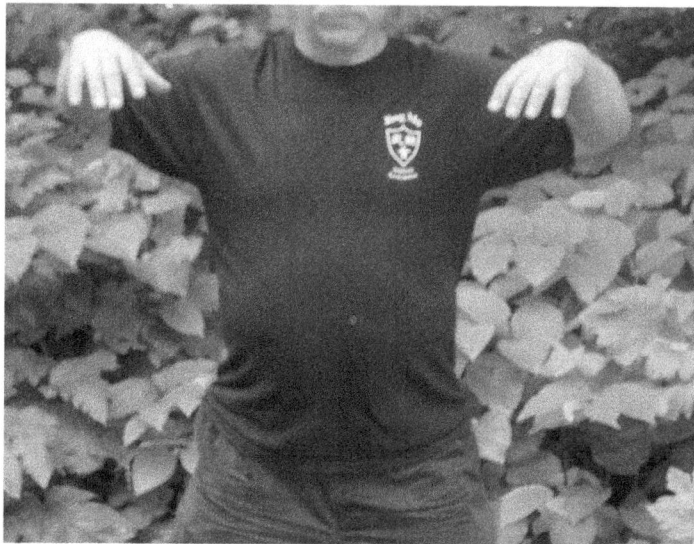

Palm outward hands are held at ear level, fingertips up, thumbs inward, at the side with elbows outward, inhale through the center of the palms.

Cradle your hips backward and downward.

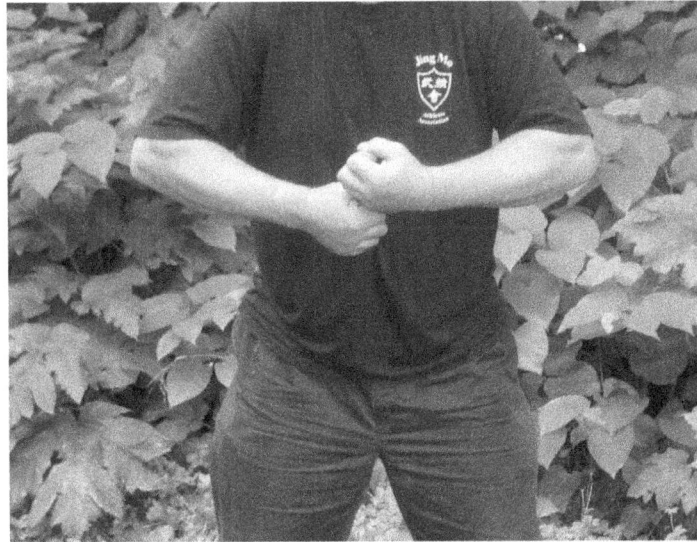

drop your elbows diagonally inward and downward to solar plexus level
as you drop your hands, changing them to palm downward,
fingertips pointing to each other and the center of the body in front:
elbows are slightly raised at the side of the torso
to about halfway at shoulder level:
on the way downward the open outstretched hands are slowly close around
the gathered energy ball at the Yongquan point, starting to wrapping it
gradually halfway in a fist;

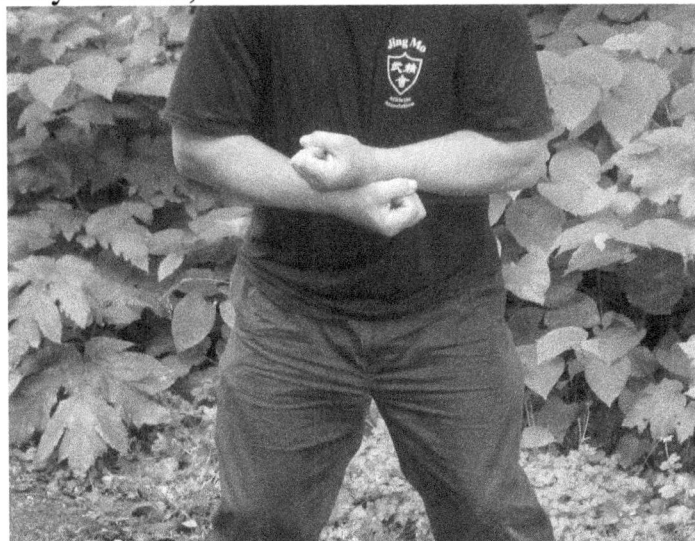

elbows are pulled inward to urge the
hands coming toward each other, with right arm underneath;

exhale and sink, as the hands cross past each other,
completely tightened into hardened fists;

after the hand pass each other tighten the fists from the abdominal area
outward to the fists, connected by the Lower Dan Tien;
gather Earth Chi from root into abdominal area,
then flow it downward through arms and legs as one sinks:
connected to the rooted Earth Chi,
cradle the hips forward and upward,
the Lower Dan Tien guides both outward fists downward,
for low level outside blocks connected to the rooted earth chi;

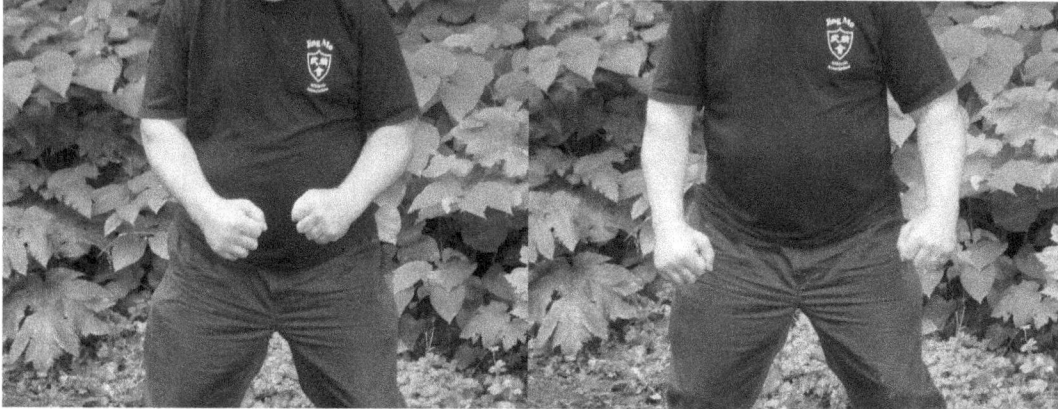

from your root, push down through the Lower Dan Tien
through the elbows,
with the widening of the knees: urge the forearms and
fists outward to inside-to-outside downward low blocks;
anchoring into the ground root.

Part 2, Upheld hands gather heaven chi into Lower Dan Tien, then one sinks:
connected to the rooted earth chi,
then the foot root pushes up through Lower Dan Tien:
which guides both upward high level inside to outside blocks.

Standing in a Horse Stance:

open-hands a held in outside-to-inside block position as before:

relax fists, and inhale as you move each hand-arm combination toward the
center, crossing them right hand over the left;

cradle the hips backward and downward.

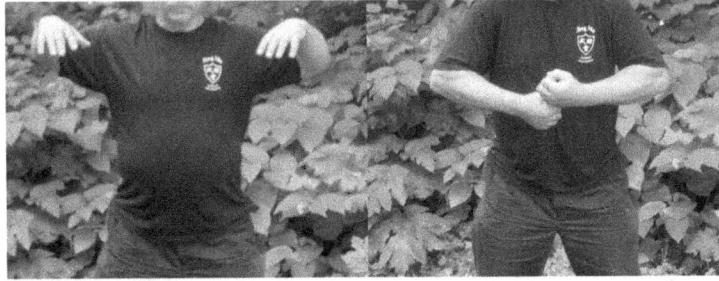

After the hand pass each other near the abdominal area,
sink your root, and drop your elbows so forearms are level,
hands will cross and go past each other at this same abdominal level, then
hands turned into loose fists:
    rotate outward to palm upward and thumb outward;
    tucked elbows urged by the Lower Dan Tien, propel the fists,
    in two simultaneous high inside to outside blocks;

tighten first from the abdominal area, then outward to the fists,
cradle the hips forward and upward,
connected at all time to the Lower Dan Tien;

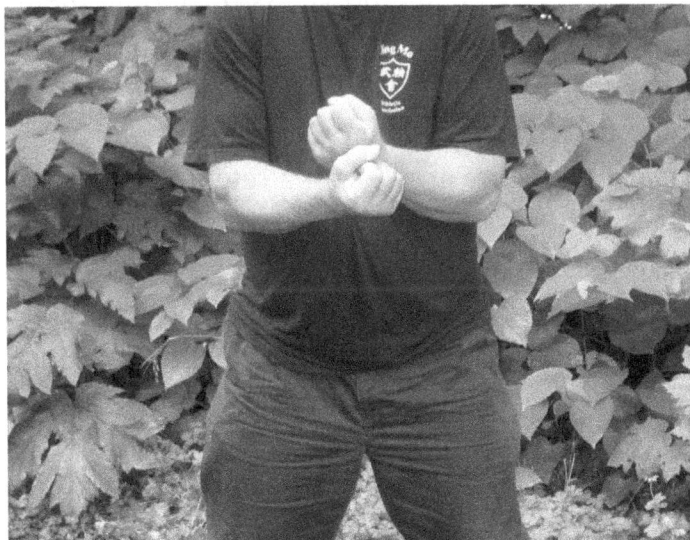

from your root, push up through the Lower Dan Tien,
the bottom of the feet move from the inside to the outside,
expanding the knees,
cradle the hip and lower buttocks area forward, in an arc;
through the elbows, urging the forearms and
fists outward to inside-to-outside blocks;
elbows tucked and lower than hands,

forearms almost act as rockers off of the tightened abdominal area, fists are palm facing, thumb outward, and extended farthest from the torso.

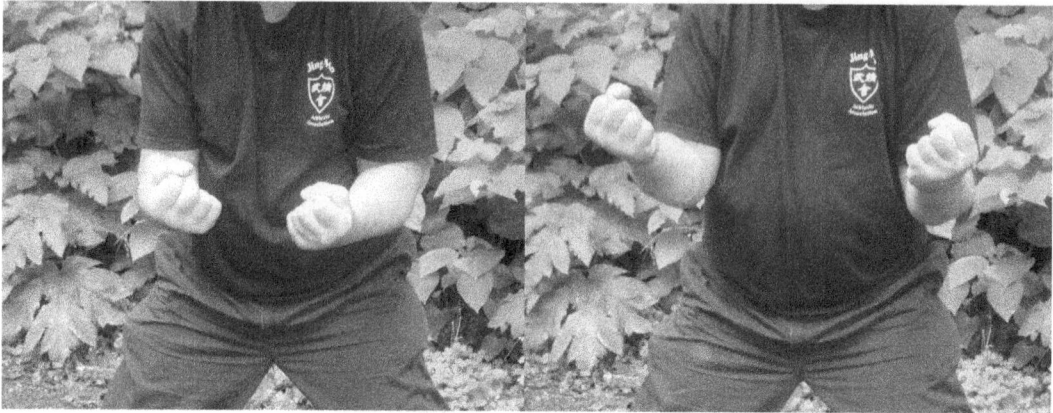

PRAYER HANDS CHI SAU

Place hands, with arms extended, in front of your Middle Dan Tien, palms facing inward 2-4 inches apart, fingertips pointing up, then:
1) move palms vertically up and down, as if rubbing them,
2) move palms in opposite circles, then change directions;
3) alternately evenly move palms
    a) closer to each other, as if compressing air;
    b) moving them further apart, as if stretching cotton candy.

TAI CHI REELING SILK

Hands move apart from their center near the Lower Dan Tien:
  a) one palm upward hand diagonally up,
  b) one palm downward moving diagonally downward,
  c) both palms moving away from each other at the same rate,
  d) the feeling between the palms is like; reeling silk out of a cocoon,
  e) the feeling on the palms is like sliding silk cloth over them.

Tai Chi, Old Super Short Form

This form is universal, as it can be practiced by any style, with it's particular accent. It was old when I studied it in the early 1970s. I have seen it used by very different schools.

The form consists of five basic moves:
1) up and down,
2) turning two arm block,
3) reeling silk to one side,
4) reeling silk to the other side, and
5) two arm press.

1) Pointing northward, bow: fist with palm.

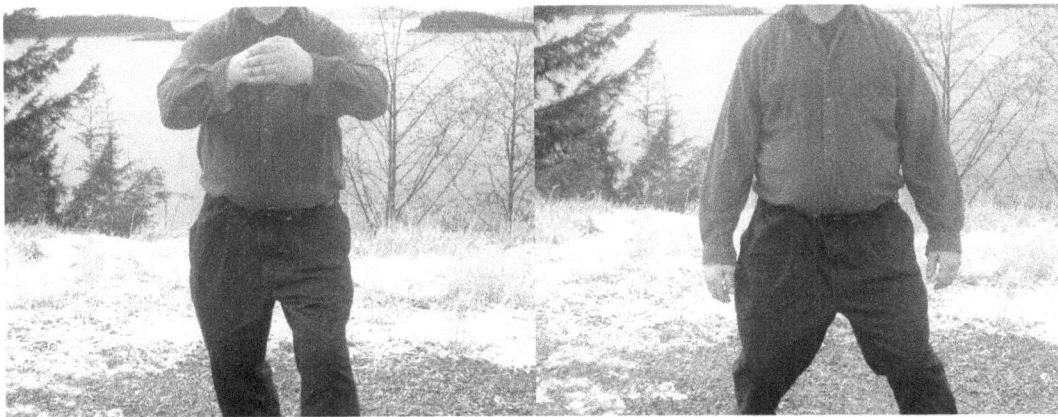

2) Left leg steps to the side into shoulder width horse stance;

    hands up and down:

    hands are at one's side,

    inhale as hands are raised,

    exhale as hands are lowered.

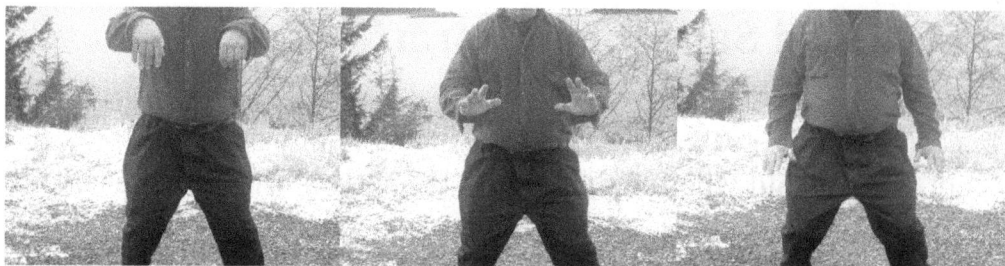

3) Up and down in place.
4) Turn to the left block:

shift weight to right leg and sink into it right leg being full, the left leg in an empty stance;

inhale as you move both hands to the right side at waist level, palms up, fingertips pointing to each other;

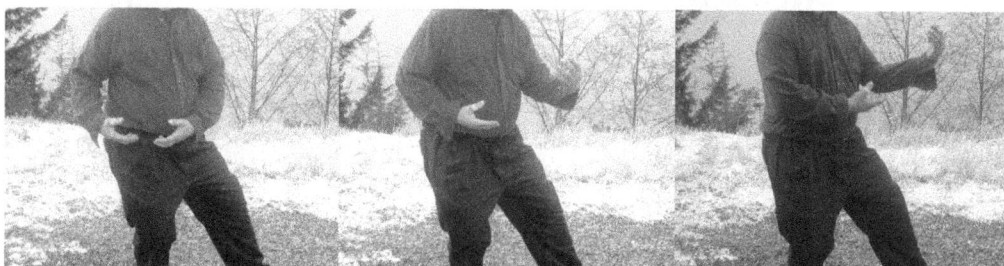

exhale as you start rotating the body toward the left by pushing with the right foot/ankle base, which moves the hips, turning and moving the left foot leftward to be at shoulder width apart and at right angle (90 degrees) to right foot;

as the body turns to the right, the turning momentum carries the arms to the left side of the body, focused by the Lower Dan Tien;

the left arms blocks from the inside upward and outward, so that it arrives fingertips upward, palm facing, with thumb on the outside, the blocking motion is a pivoting at the left elbow, with the forearm being swung from the elbow, that rests at waist level;

the right arm performs a lower-than-waist block by pivoting on the elbow base near the waist to move the right forearm inward toward the left: blocking with ridge hand at waistline, or heel hand for lower attack;

both arms are primarily moved by the rotation of the body.

5) Reeling Silk to the Right:

both hands drop to waist level on the left side, as if holding a ball, left hand on top with palm downward, right hand on bottom, palm upward;

inhale and sink slightly bending at the knees, as you gather Chi in between your palms, this is the ball held like a cup of water between your side and center;

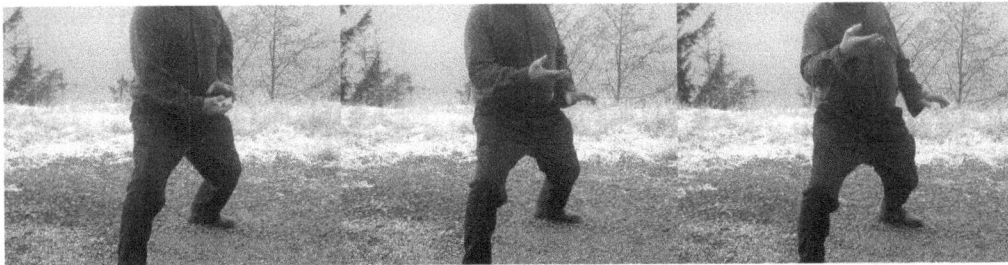

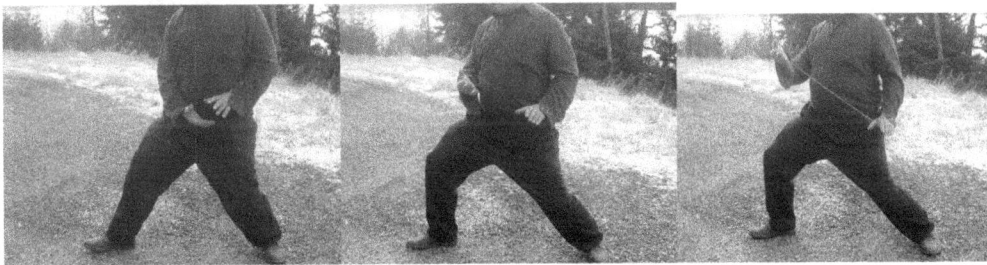

exhale as you move both arms simultaneously away from each other, on a diagonal plane of 45 degrees or less: the front right ridge palm upward hand sliding upward, as the rear left heel ridge palm downward hand slides downward;

this is the action of reeling the silk from a silk worm's cocoon, in order to draw out the silk successfully the action must be consistent and smoothly; without jerking or changing direction sharply (when done too fast the silk breaks; when too slow, it sticks to itself and becomes tangled);

the connection between the two palms could also be viewed as salt water taffy: bending and stretching, but not tearing;

the Chi between your hands is shared and separated evenly between the two hands.

6) Reeling Silk to the Left.

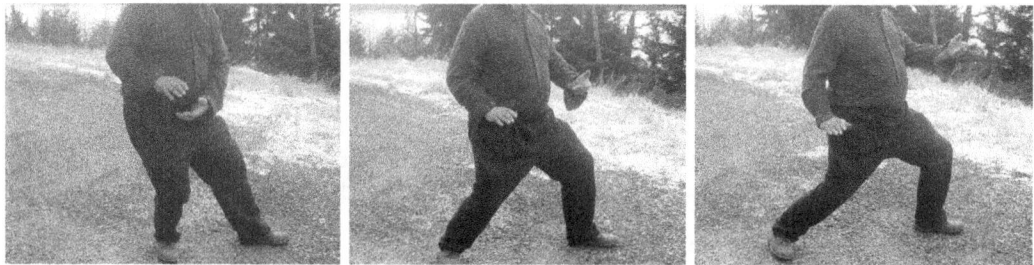

7) Two handed press, left side:

prayer-hands near left shoulder:

inhale, as both hands are held fingertips up, palms facing each other with a small gap in between hands as if holding a ball, gap between hands is 4 – 8 inches;

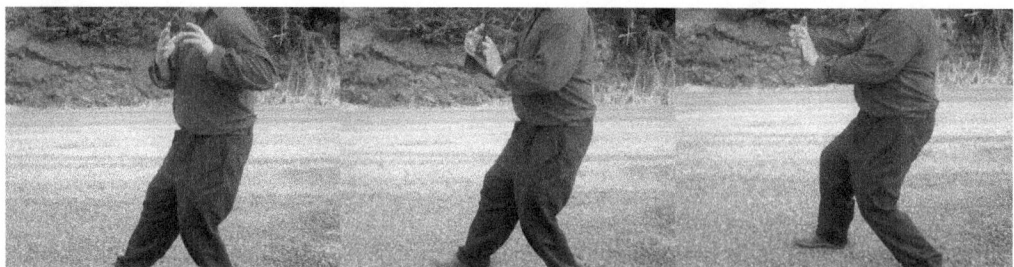

slowly start to exhale, as you move prayer hands from left shoulder to center of body, in front of Middle Dan Tien, as you rotate left hand in front, to be pointed horizontally rightward and move rearward and rotate right hand fingertips upward, palm outward;

start to sink into the rear left leg, increasing the exhalation as you squeeze the rear left foot's ankle to push your midsection forward;

as the hand pair is lead straight horizontally forward by Lower Dan Tien, the gap between the hands is decreased to 0 to 2 inches apart, the rear right hand projecting through and combing with the front left hand.

8) Right leg steps up to even horse stance, up and down with hands.

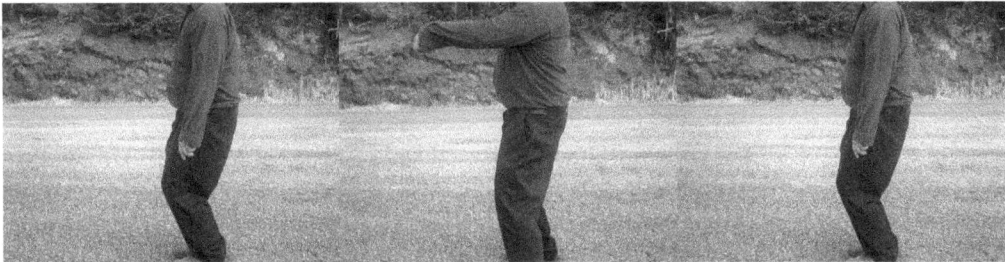

9) Left leg together with right; up and down in place, then bow, which should point you eastward.

To continue; repeat steps 2-9,
for 3 more times,
to end up where you started.

Do four repetitions in the opposite direction.

Kung Fu, Old Super Short Form

1) Pointing northward, bow: fist with palm.
2) Left leg steps to the side into shoulder width horse stance;

    hands up and down:

    hands are at one's side,

    inhale as hands are raised,

    exhale as hands are lowered.

3) Up and down in place.
4) Turn to the left block:

    shift weight to right leg and sink into it right leg being full, the left leg in an empty stance;

    inhale as you move both hands to the right side at waist level, palms up, fingertips pointing to each other;

    exhale as you start rotating the body toward the left by pushing with the right foot/ankle base, which moves the hips, turning and moving the left foot leftward to be at shoulder width apart and at right angle (90 degrees) to right foot;

    as the body turns to the right, the turning momentum carries the arms to the left side of the body, focused by the Lower Dan Tien;

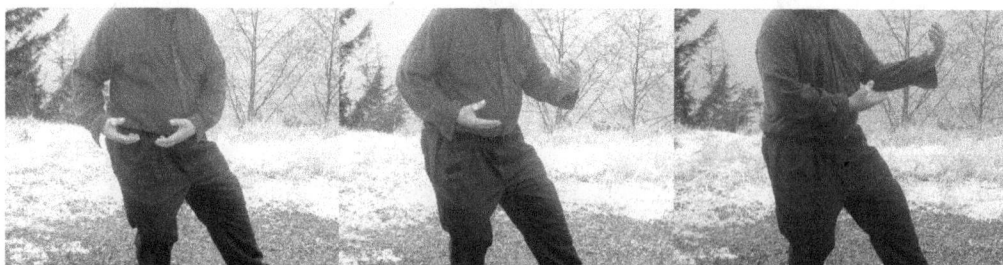

the left arms blocks from the inside upward and outward, so that it arrives fingertips upward, palm facing, with thumb on the outside, the blocking motion is a pivoting at the left elbow, with the forearm being swung from the elbow, that rests at waist level;

the right arm performs a lower-than-waist block by pivoting on the elbow base near the waist to move the right forearm inward toward the left: blocking with ridge hand at waistline, or heel hand for lower attack;

both arms are primarily moved by the rotation of the body.

5) High mantis/crane-hand block to the right with right hand, while left hand does inside ridge-hand high then low block sweep:

inhale and sink slightly bending at the knees, as you gather the left hand is moving toward your Lower Dan Tien and the right hand, Chi is between your hands, this is the ball held like a cup of water between your side and center;

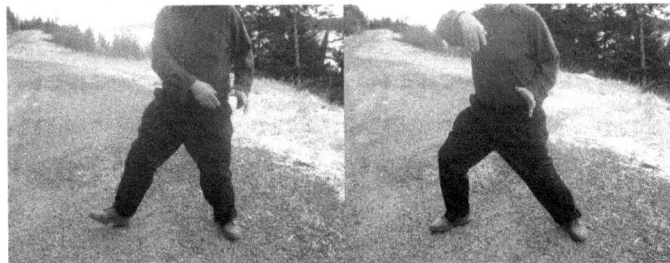

as you start the shifting of the body rightward by angling the left ankle, then knee to urge the right foot to turn on it's heel outward to the right followed by the right knee;

the left forearm rotates inward at elbow for outside to inside high block, simultaneously rotate the right forearm upward at the elbow;

start the exhale as the downward sweeping left arm past the being - level with the ground, the fingertips will pass by the right palm: arms are moving away from each other and your center;

left forearm continues low inside to outside sweeping block downward, simultaneously right hand turns to mantis/crane hand blocking upward and sideward as a deflecting mantis/crane block, using end of the forearm; when blocking higher, up to head high; continue upward and backward;

the Chi between your hands is shared and separated evenly between the two hands, usually focused at the point of the block/strike.

6) High mantis/crane-hand block to the left with left hand, while inside ridge-hand does low block sweep with right hand.

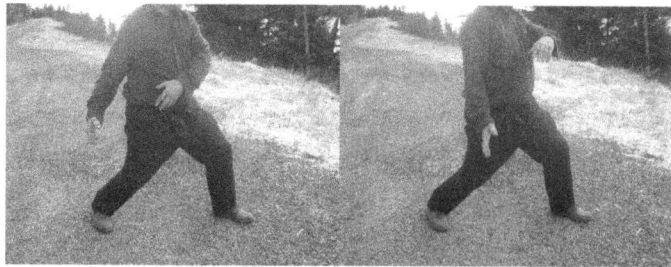

A combination of 5) and 6) is one circular cycle pattern, the length of the swirling arms is determined by how much they are bent. One can use this pattern as a continuous and returning fist to trap all incoming strikes, until an opening is apparent, then deliver 7) reinforced back-fist.

7) Reinforce right handed back-fist to head:

 prayer-hands near left shoulder:

inhale, as both hands are held fingertips up, palms facing each other with a small gap in between hands as if holding a ball, gap between hands is 4 – 8 inches;

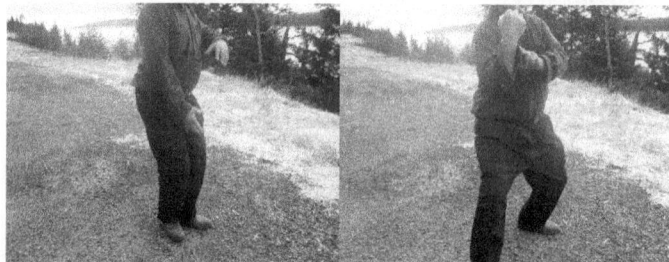

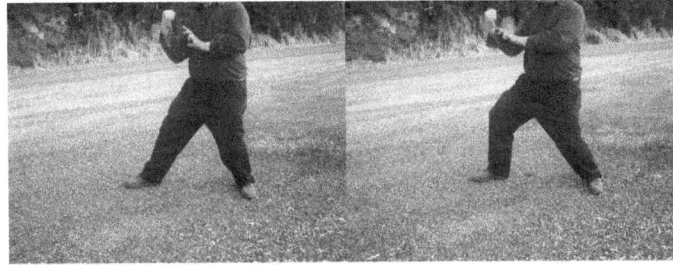

slowly start to exhale, as you move prayer hands from left shoulder to center of body, in front of Middle Dan Tien, as you rotate left hand in front, to be pointed horizontally rightward and move rearward and rotate right hand fingertips upward, palm outward;

start to sink into the rear left leg, increasing the exhalation as you squeeze the rear left foot's ankle to push your midsection forward;

as the hand pair is lead straight horizontally forward by Lower Dan Tien, the gap between the hands is decreased to 0 to 2 inches apart, the rear right hand projecting through and combing with the front left hand.

7) Right leg steps up to even horse stance, up and down with hands.
8) Left leg together with right; up and down in place, then bow, which should point you eastward.

To continue; repeat steps 2-8,
for 3 more times,

to end up where you started.

Do four repetitions in the opposite direction.

FOREARM THROW: Developing Sensitivity of Opponent's Root, Center of Qi, Balance and Root

A prerequisite is to be familiar with the Rowing Exercise (page 49), Shifting the Water (page 46) or equivalent.
This is a four part exercise:
  1) arm swinging in-place,
  2) step and turn 180 degrees while swinging arms from side to side,
  3) step and turn with a staff,
  4) step and turn with a partner using a throw or arm-lock.

1) Arm Swing Side To Side

  a) Stand in a Horse Stance with both arms hanging relaxed at the left side of your waist. Next our arms will be moving from the left side to the right side.

  b) Left side should be full (of Qi and usually more weighted) and right side empty, left leg slightly more bent than right.
  Movement will start at ankle, continue through the knee, then hip and directed by the Lower Dan Tien.
  Inhale while raising both arms simultaneously to shoulder level to midpoint at center in front of you; as you open your palms to face outward, fingertips pointing upward.

  c) Exhale and sink, as your arms swing continues past midpoint, allowing your hands to relax and arms to drop to the right side near your waist. Left side becomes empty as arms move past midpoint and right side becomes full as arms continue to the right side of the waist, sinking your stance.

  Repeat a) b) and c) from the right side to left side.

  Practice this till you can raise your arms with your breath and waist/hip-movement, rather than using muscle. It will help to inhale through your opening palms; as they raise to the shoulder-level midpoint.

2) Step and Turn 180 Degrees While Swinging Arms
   (arms swing up and out from side to side while stepping forward
   and doing a half turn)

a) Stand in a T-Stance right leg extended feet pointed directly in front of
   you, left leg pointed toward the left side; feet at right angle.
   Arms hang loosely at left side.

   Turn your right foot outward to the right, by rotating it at the heel.
   Left side is full and right side is empty, right foot is empty.
   Two-thirds of the weight is on the rear left foot.

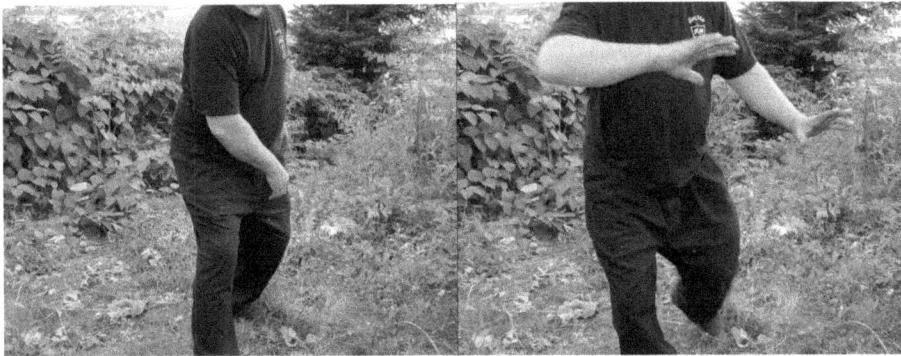

b) Right foot is slid a little forward in an empty step.
   Right foot is turned outward on the heel.

c) Arms are swung from the left side at hip, slightly upward to midpoint
   at shoulder level.

d) As the arms cross your center line, they carry you forward and to the right while you pivot 180 degrees on your front right foot.

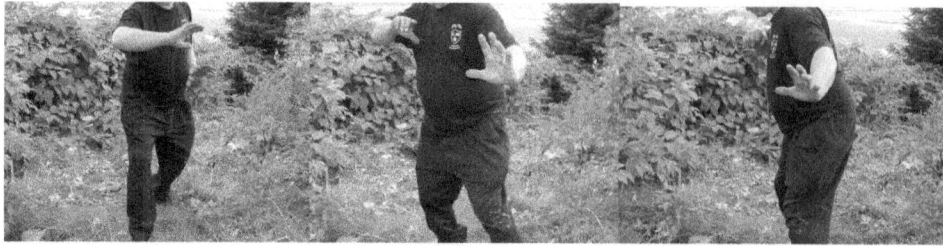

e) As the arms cross your center line, they carry you forward and to the right while you pivot 180 degrees on your now left new front foot.

f) You complete the spin by landing on your now right new rear foot, sinking on this back leg, bending it slightly and dropping your arms at your right side at waist level.

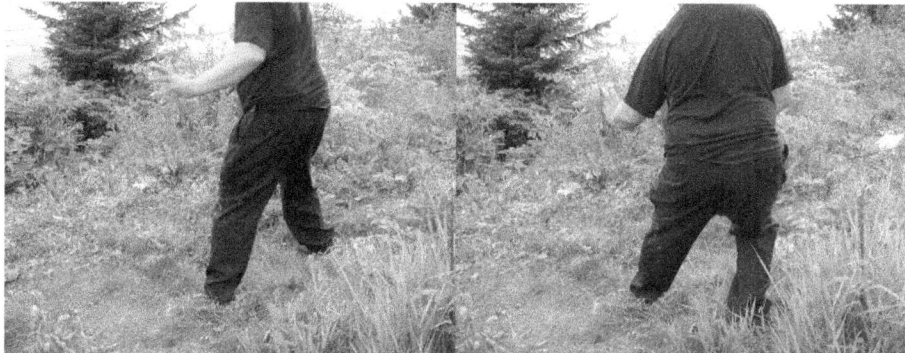

g) Repeat process a) through e) but on opposite sides, and then you will return back where you started from. Inhale on the way up to the center midpoint, exhaling past the center as you sink to the opposite side.

3) Step and Turn with a Staff
   (staff drawn and swung upward and out, from side to side while stepping forward and doing a half turn)

a) Stand in a T-Stance right leg extended feet pointed directly in front of you, left leg pointed toward the left side; feet at right angle.
   Staff angled downward at left side, right hand on the top two-thirds section, left hand on the bottom third section of the staff.

It is helpful to view the staff as a pipe half-full of water, with the water filled on the bottom of the pipe, the top half of the pipe being empty.

Turn your right foot outward to the right, by rotating it at the heel. Left side is full and right side is empty, right foot is empty. Two-thirds of the weight is on the rear left foot.

b) Right foot is slid a little forward in an empty step.
Right foot is turned outward on the heel.

Staff is drawn as a sword and swung from the left side at hip, slightly upward to midpoint at shoulder level. It is helpful to view the staff as a pipe half full of water, with the water occupying the pipe evenly, or at midpoint.

As the staff crosses your center line, it and your momentum carry you forward and to the right; while you pivot 180 degrees on your right front foot. It is helpful to view the staff as a pipe half full of water, with the water moving from the left side to the right side, as it crosses the midpoint at shoulder level.

c) You complete the spin by landing on your now left rear foot, sinking on this back leg, bending it slightly and dropping the staff to your right side at waist level. The staff view as a pipe half full of water, shifts to the other side of the pipe, with the water filled on the bottom of the pipe, the top half of the pipe being empty.

Repeat process a) through c) but on the opposite side, with staff angled downward at right side, left hand on the top two-thirds section, right hand on the bottom third section of the staff; this will return you back to where you started from. Inhale on the way up to the center midpoint, exhaling past the center as you sink to the opposite side.

4) Step and Turn with a Partner
(arms swing up and out from side to side while stepping forward and doing a half turn, then pulling opponent down, up and circling their captured arms in a circle; throwing the opponent)

Opponent/practicing-partner stands facing you with their right arm fully extended with a front punch, their right foot forward in a bow stance (a longer length-wise extended T-stance expanded to width-wise to shoulder width; 2/3 weight on back leg).

a) Stand in a T-Stance right leg extended, right foot pointed directly in front of you, left leg pointed toward the left side; feet at right angle. Arms hang loosely at waist-level left side.
   Turn your right foot outward to the right, by rotating it at the heel.
   Left side is full and right side is empty, right foot is empty.
   Two-thirds of the weight is on the rear left foot.
b) Right foot is slid a little forward in an empty step.
   Right foot is turned outward on the heel.
c) Arms are swung from the left side at hip, slightly upward to midpoint at shoulder level.
d) As the arms cross your center line, grab the opponent's right arm forward punch's outside wrist with your right hand.
e) Use the momentum of your swing and the grab (or sticking); to carry you forward as you left hand grabs (or checks) the opponent's right arm at the elbow.
f) If opponent is rigid and stationary, the left hand continues through for an arm break.
g) Other-wise and you pivot 180 degrees on your front right foot.
h) If opponent is coming forcefully and well rooted forward, you do a half-spin around them.
i) Option f) again or you spin just far enough to be slightly behind them, pulling their right arm to full extension, uprooting them, and continue to a complete your 180 degree spin.
j) While still holding opponent's captured right arm, sink back ward into a T-stance or bow stance in reverse of your starting position;
   left leg extended feet pointed directly in front of you, right leg pointed toward the left side; feet at right angle.

j) As you sink into your rear leg pull opponent's arm downward and you, by bending you rear knee first, and continue the pull with your Lower Dan Tien pulling you arms and his.

k) Circle the arm pair clockwise, with an option of releasing opponent at completion to be thrown.

Start drill with opponent's right arm stationary, and they are not moving, next with the opponent striking slowly.

Proceed to the opponent moving forward with their punch.
Rigid arm practices should not be practiced by beginners or someone will end up accidentally breaking their partner's arm.

When both partners have learned the above, the opponent can resist more; but confine their resisting to mutually agreed upon points in the swing, and throw. This will require that the throwing partner be familiar with Chi Na, for throwing and locking options that were facilitated by this side-stepping catch and spin.

CHINESE SPEAR

Under the guise of warfare, the British in the mid-nineteenth century concluded that the Chinese spear was far superior to their bayonets. Currently, the weapon is smaller and its uses are compressed into about thirty different methods.

Some of the famous spear exercises are from the Stone family; the Horse family; the Yang family, and the Northern Shaolin system.

The spear is generally taught after the student has obtained a firm understanding of the staff. It is the ideal weapon for the student whose physical characteristics are agility and speed. In the hands of an expert, the execution of a spear can be considered to be nearly invincible.

Regardless of the martial arts systems, spear techniques are designed to teach the principles and the importance of fluidity, grace (smoothness), good balance, precision-based attack, and defense techniques. With proper practice, the quickness and overall agility of the spear player can be enhanced.

While the Chinese straight sword is considered to be the most difficult to learn, the spear is considered to be the next most difficult of all Chinese weapons to master. In the same manner of the straight sword, the proper execution of the spear can also improve the concentration of the practitioner.

Due to its history and its lethal but proficient techniques, the spear has been nicknamed The Emperor of All Chinese Long Weapons. During ancient China, some spear forms were practiced on a horse.

When utilizing a spear in combat, it is important that one should never move the spear too far away from the center line of the torso.

The main purpose of learning to use a spear is to build power by learning correct body methods (Shenfa) to open up the joints and dynamically stretches the tendons. This method must be used to improve one's skill. People, that do not practice martial arts or do not practice it correctly, will have rather stiff joints that limit their range of movements. With proper long spear practice, one can open the joints, increase flexibility, and therefore improve agility of movements. Some spear sets emphasize subtle wrist and waist movements that can emit powerful circular movements, which can be technically lethal in combat.

Every time the spear moves the tip should vibrate. The more the staff vibrates, or appears to be flexible: the more the Chi has been generated and directed to the killing end.

This is not the same as using the leverage of the heavier spear end like a whip. Chi should be generated from the Lower Dan Tien.

CHINESE LONG STAFF

An easier Staff set **Fire - Water Staff Fighting** then
Ground Demon Staff

The hands should slide up and down the staff and should end up 12 inches apart upon each strike; with one hand holding the very end of the staff (Yang Position) and 12 inches away the other hand is positioned in the Yin position. Most people cannot generate the power with the hands only 12 inches apart so we see them with their hands 20 - 24 inches apart.

The more the staff vibrates, or appears to be flexible: the more the Chi has been generated and directed to the killing end.

Every time the staff moves the tip of the staff should vibrate.

See more under **Hsing-i Spear, in the Hsing-i Workouts Chapter**, page 133.

POWER

Chinese method to express power is not largely based on using muscular strength; a point, which can be compared to hitting a nail on the head with a hammer. If the angle is not aligned perfectly with the nail, the blow will be deflected and the nail bent. If the strike is not controlled, it will not drive the nail, it will be incorrectly pushed.

One of the best methods for developing **Fa Jing**, is mentioned in Robert Smith's book, Chinese Boxing, Masters and Methods:
stand in the Hsing-i San Ti stance, and do the element Metal, holding the pose near the end of the strike, for three breaths.

A straight piece of straw can be driven into solid oak, by tornadoes.
This says a lot about a true and effective strike.

For a firm root, best to hold the San Ti stance for an hour plus.

ROOTING

When one is born, they will normally move internally, up to the age of around two years. An experiment for one to try; is to put a coin, or small object in an infants palm, and let him close his hand around it. If the infant wants to hold that coin, a grown man will have difficulty opening the infant's hand. If this was due to muscular strength, there would be no contest. The infant is using Qi (Chi), something that we are all born with.

As the years go, the child will learn how to move, from humans, whereas his first moves are intrinsic, primal, and natural. From humans, he learns that you are supposed to use your muscles and bones, this way and that, and looses his unfiltered unprocessed, indescribable ability.

Throwing a punch uses different muscles groupings in the arm. A child might take up boxing, where he will learn to use the right muscles in his arm, and shoulders. In karate, and the better boxing schools, and Judo; he will learn to use his hips. From there he might be content to refine these abilities, switch to the internal, or use both external and internal.

The internal will start with the flow of energy, and the lack of tension in the muscles. For general health purposes, this might be enough. For martial purposes, and for dealing with forces greater than oneself, they may be able to connect this energy flow of chi, to their Lower Dan Tien (just below the navel area).

It is highly advantageous, to connect this to, or below the ground, your root (hence foundation). This use of the ground is ironically, is most highly developed in Hsing-i, but is also employed by the better warrior/fighters of Shotokan, Goju, Shto Ryu, and Tae Kwon Do, in their step-stomp punch.

A crude mechanical comparison, would be of a car coming to an intersection, applying its brakes, and something getting hit by the car, as it stretches forward, after the brakes are applied. This is a good example of the Ying/Yang theory, of something becoming so extreme, that it becomes its opposite. Predominately hard and external Shotokan etc., at the highest levels becomes so hard, that it become soft, so external, that it eventually become internal (usually not taught till 2nd degree and up).

Some methods for strengthening your stance:

1) The extreme of full Riding Horse stance, is sinking until your thighs are parallel to the ground, and then balancing a tea cup on your thigh.

2) Holding a stance for 30-60 minutes.

3) Stand in your stance, near a railroad track, on a trestle or a bridge and see how balanced, centered, and low you can go; as the train passes by.

4) Stand in your stance, and root, or move in your set slowly, while atop a boat deck, raft, or small shaky floating pier.

5) An external way of developing a good Qi (Chi) root, is to hike a while uphill, with a pack of 50-100% of your body weight.

6) Barefoot water skiing.

7) Being pulled with a rope by a car or tractor through the sand, shoe-skiing.

8) Skriing (starting a small rockslide and riding it down the mountain..

9) Have a partner stand on your thighs or shoulders, while you are in a horse stance.

10) Pushing or pulling a car by foot.

A Martial Artist stance without rooting, is like a house, without a foundation.

A few internal exercises to develop and check this root, are:

1) Stand in your stance, near a railroad track, on a trestle or a bridge and see how balanced, centered, and low you can go, as the train passes by.
2) Stand in your stance, and root, or move in your set slowly, while atop a boat deck, raft, or small shaky floating pier.

In both of these exercises, try going front to back, left to right, and get a 'rock the cradle' cadence going. It is easier to exhale, as you sink and or retreat, and inhale as you rise, and/or advance.

An external way of developing a good Chi root, is to hike a while up hill, with a pack of 50-100% of your body wait. Do your sets, Rowing Exercises (page 49), or the Tai Chi posture Standing Pole - Embrace the Moon, (page 41), after you have gone as far as you can.

A Martial Art without rooting, is like a house, without a foundation. There are many techniques, and meditations for developing grounding, and/or one's root, some of these involve meditation, and/or Qi Gong (Chi Kung).

The following are some methods that are not widely taught, but are effective. This is not an attempt to replace those techniques, and/or styles, only to add to them.

Bare handed cliff climbing.

Running at night.

Running in the woods.

Running on railroad tracks.

Running up stairs.

Hiking uphill with a pack 50-100% of your body weight.

Doing the Tai Chi posture Standing Pole (Embrace the Moon) for an hour.

Starting a workout of 3 hours+ by doing 100 repetitions of every kick, for a total of 1,000 kicks each leg, then proceeding to forms etc.

Power squats, with few repetitions, so as not to overly wear out the knees.

Having a classmate stand on your shoulders or waist: while you are in a stance.

Doing your forms in sand: till you sink.

Sea Legs: doing your forms on a boat or raft (from the Old Salt School).

Marathon running cross country trails.

Cross-country skiing uphill: for long distances.

Walking Ba Gua style; on smooth ice.

Doing the Tai-Chi position Embrace the Moon, while emphasizing the flow of the Earth Chi, coming from 6 inches to 6 feet below your feet, coming up through the soles, channeled by the lower Dan Tien to the arms and fingers. The space between the hands should be paid attention to, since it is like the gap of a spark plug, or the brushes of an electric motor.

The 'minds eye' should be oriented toward the center of the body. "After the whole body is relaxed, the mind must also be relaxed, but be slightly oriented to the navel (the center of the body or Lower Dan Tien). It must be noted that slight orientation means that the mind must not be excessively oriented; otherwise the result may be just to the contrary. Nervous tension may result from it. In serious cases such un-wholesome results as the over-tension of the nerves; may even be created." from a Pa Tuan Ching classic.

You will learn to see yourself, and it will be unnecessary to theorize, it will be unneeded to secure this information from someone else. As long as you rely on someone else's advise, it will be external, by definition.

To see/feel one's insides is internal. To explain or understand it; is not.

HSING-I STEP METHOD

Advance by stepping low, step high when retreating. When starting the step, the toe grinds the ground and the heel rises up, the foot takes a flowing step.

When moving the body, the step is of first importance. The step is the root of the body, it is the central axis of motion. Since the whole body is used in an encounter with an enemy, the person who wishes to be unbeatable must rely on the handwork, but it is the footwork that allows the hands to adapt and change to the advantageous position. Advancing, retreating, turning or angling, without the steps; how can one have a chance? Lowering, rising, extending or contracting, without footwork; how can one execute profound changes?

To close the gap between the opponent with a forward sliding step, keeping the rear leg firmly rooted,: 1) the front leg moves in curves, snaking into the best position and 2) roots, and then the 3) rear leg empties root and slides with the front leg's advance forward and re-roots to drive the 4) front foot 's angling (sometimes sliding forward a little), to go with forward force; changing to mid-length sinking San Ti stance. This is an in-place shuffle.

The saying is that the eyes are key and the heart decides the reaction, in all changes and turns of the body, in reaction to all types of affront, it must be that footwork is the leader. In addition, the steps must not be forced. Movement must spring from an empty heart, as if dancing without conscious effort, the body desires to move and steps turn to all sides. The hands are about to move, the steps also urge them in motion. Without timing it so, it is so; without making it go, it goes; this is what is referred to as the upper wishes to move and the lower follows.

Those who do not put the body and foot work first in importance; will not be successful in defeating enemies. This must not be taken lightly.

Come with a scissors step, the legs move in a scissors motion. Move the steps by inches. Advance with low steps, retreat with high steps. It is important to have the correct sequence of movement, dodging, or leaping about; the feet follow. Using the feet to strike, the intent to stomp never misses, the feeling completely relies on the snapping of the rear foot. Keep feeling in the rear foot, and advance attacking with a stomping strike that shows no mercy.

If the hands are raised without the feet rising; it is also a waste of time; if the feet are raised, but the hands are not raised, it is again a waste of time. If separated by a distance of ten feet, the steps must be fast, two heads turning, the most important is the inch step. Step straight in between the opponent's legs, drill in through his crotch.

The front leg relies on the back leg, the rear steps down to the ankle; the rear leg relies on the front leg, the ankle is raised in sequence.

In regards to step methods; there are inch steps, fast steps, and stomping steps; none must be omitted. In regards to leg work, there is lifting and drilling, lowering and overturning; not drilling nor overturning. The most important is the inch step. The feet are seventy percent and the hands are thirty percent. The leg step into the opponent's center and steals his position.

The movements originate from *no heart* with *no intention* and the excitement is generated from *no feeling.* When the body wishes to move, the stepping will also move around automatically. When the hands are going to move, you have already stepped to the opponent's key position. This happens (naturally) without expectation, progresses without being pushed. This is called; the top wishes to move the bottom naturally follows.

Stepping is divided into front leg and rear leg; such as the front leg steps forward, the rear leg will follow. The front and the rear all have a definite position.

Doing Hsing-i going downhill; will also help correct the front foot placement and accent.

To feel something before a person moves. This a non-physical manifestation of a physical one, but not a mental thought.

Perhaps there is something to be said about the gray area between Consciousness and Form, in the process of consciousness creating form.

Crows know this, for when you have hunting one on your mind, none will be found.

HSING-I MIND

Xing, the shape of imitating combines with Yi, the mind generated from the Xin (heart); to be Xing Yi (Hsing-i)

This is to say that Yi, the wisdom mind, is generated from the emotional mind; Xin. Xin is the first mind, its characteristics are excitable and agile, whereas Yi is calm, clear and accurate.

Man has a Ling (supernatural spirit). He is able to feel and respond to everything. This is because he has a Xin (emotional mind) internally to comprehend the surrounding objects. Objects are external but the comprehending is internal.

When the Xin (emotional mind) is steady, the Shen (spirit) is calm. When the Shen is calm, the Xin is peaceful. When the Xin is peaceful, it is quite and clean. When it is quite and clean, then nothing exists. When nothing exists, the Qi will be moved smoothly. When Qi is transported smoothly, then the imagination disappears. When the feeling is clear, then the Shen and Qi are mutually connected. Qi returns to its roots.

The three Yi's must be linked together means; Xin Yi, Qi Yi, and the Li Yi must be connected into one. This is what is called the three internal connections. Among the three, the Xin is the planner, the Qi is the marshal, and the Li (strength) is the generals and soldiers.

If the Qi is not full, then the Li will not be sufficient. Although the Xin has the plan, it is still in vain (i.e., empty). When the Qi and Yi are trained well, then the marshal is able to use Yi to control Li and correspond internally with the Xin Yi. In the connections of these three Yis, the Qi must be especially the first concern.

When you train, the Xin should not be alarmed and hasty. When alarmed, you have the Yi of fright and fear. When you are hasty, then you have the Yi of the fast and abrupt. When you are frightened, then the Qi must be weak. When you are weak and disordered: the movement of the hands and feet are not manageable. The Xin must be leisurely; so as not to be hasty or scared. In fact, this corresponds with the Qi externally and internally.

The eyes must be venomous; acute, sharp and stern, with a mean and serious look.

A major difference of Hsing-i, is that the first mind, the so-called emotional mind, Xing, is not to be suppressed, rather it is cultivated since Xing Yi imitates the animal form, mind and spirit. In some other internal martial arts, and Qi Gong; the emotional mind is suppressed and dominated by Yi, the wisdom mind.

This emotional mind is the fastest, as it is travels from the thalamus, then to the amygdale.

The renown researcher of the neurology of fear, Dr. Joseph DeLoux of New York University, in his book The Emotional Brain, found that there are two kinds of fear in the brain: fast fear and slow fear.

Fast fear travels the low road of the brain: senses to thalamus, then to the amygdale, which is located deep within the brain on the temporal sides; time 12 milliseconds. Traditional philosophy represents this separation as horse mind (slow) controlling the monkey mind (fast).

Slow fear travels the high road of the brain: senses to thalamus which sends it to the cortex (higher up); time 24 milliseconds.

Both systems occur simultaneously, with the same sense data, the theory being that you cannot have speed and accuracy on the same circuit.

Bear in mind, this is not the time to process the information, or physically move to react.

12 milliseconds or 1 hundredth of a second might not seem like much difference, but consider that there are some people that can beat a flash. Beating a flash is blinking your eyes when a photo is shot with a flash. The difference in speed between the flash, and camera shutter is one fiftieth of a second, or 2 hundredths. I and others can beat it trying, and by surprise, some just by surprise. Memory and choice have to go to the cortex, so they are slower; test your reaction theory with the flash.

This can not be reached through force or from imitating. When it is time to be calm, it is quite and transparent. In this position, you are steady like a mountain. When it is time to move, move like thunder and like a mountain collapsing. The speed of emitting (Jin) is like lighting.

When calm; nothing is not calm. The surface and the internal, the top and the bottom; all without disorder and the meaning of inhibiting each other . When moving, nothing does not move. The left and the right, the front and the rear: all without pulling and the shape of swiftly moving around. It is just like water flowing downward; so powerful that nothing is able to stop it. It is like a canon is fired internally. Without considering thinking, without bothering to plan, simply reach the goal without expectation.

This is Hsing-Yi's highest level of achievement: the mind is mindless; you do nothing and have done everything. In the emptiness we find prenatal bodies. But do not be overly concerned about this. If you try too hard, it will elude you. Instead of trying to achieve it, pretend you already have it. This will help your mind. After all, the mind is the embodiment of your actions: therefore, Hsing-Yi is mind boxing.

'To master Hsing Yi, your mind must be empty. Start with an empty mind and imagine yourself bodiless. Although you have a mind, imagine yourself mindless. An old sage said, "Mindless mind, insubstantial-substantial." If you are attacked, counter naturally. Hit the person as if you were disembodied. You come to be the same as a Taoist: mind, mindless; body, bodiless; something, nothing.' From Liu Ch'i-Lan

The stable, calm, wisdom mind (Yi), originates from the quick, unstable, emotional, heart-mind (Xin). It is associated with the horse, whereas Xin is thought of as monkey mind;   In combining Yi and Xin; movements are fast and accurate, yet precise and calm. Qigong the emotional mind is not used, but in Hsing-i it is used to excite the spirit and be closer to the animal state, in general.

The heart moves like fire rising,
The liver moves like an arrow flying.
The spleen moves the Qi to consolidate like a ball.
The lungs move with the sound of thunder.
The kidneys move like lightning dodging.

MEDITATION

While I was studying with a Martial Arts Master, we were practicing, and he walking among us when a bumble bee flew by, the instructor, Mo Duk Kwan Master Kenny Yuen, had grabbed it by the tip of its wing. He held it there momentarily, and then released it unharmed, and the bumble bee flew off.

A bumble bees wings are fragile yet move at over 100 miles per hour and are beating in a very small wing space pattern; that moves with flight.

We asked how did he do it and the master replied that he did not 'do it', he was just there. He did not try; it was not so much being quick, as being one with the timing. One normally cannot do this without meditation.

Before meditating, it is good to clear the mind of distractions, by a method most comfortable with you, reflecting on what has been done that day, what needs to be done, then putting it aside;

Four vows/basics of Buddhism:
sentient beings are numberless, I take a vow to save them;
the deluding passions are inexhaustible, I take a vow to destroy them;
the Gates of Dharma are manifold, I take a vow to enter them;
the Buddha way is supreme, I take a vow to complete it.

Some other options for clearing the mind before meditation are; paying respect to the Four Directions, lighting a candle or piece of incense, or a general well being type of prayer such as the Lord's Prayer. Any prayer or preparation will do fine as long as it is not asking for anything specific, and does not overly tax the mind. This clears the air.

For meditation, a relaxed posture is recommended, that is stable and comfortable; usually kneeling or cross-legged.

Now regulate your breath, inhaling and holding it for as long as comfortable, then exhale, and hold it for the same amount of time. This is the foundation of the basic meditation.

When you exhale, relax the anus area (Gu Dao or Huyin Point); as you inhale, lift up the anus area.

The first concept of meditation, is usually the concept of *No Thing*. Not nothing, zero or blanks proper, but the absence of things. Every thing has some *no thing* in it, and come from being *no thing*. An expert might know a lot about one thing, but if he thinks that this makes him an expert at all things, he is mistaken, and does not know anything, since he thinks that his something, is everything. This kind of person, will give advise on something, whether he knows about it or not, so his advise cannot be trusted.

A wise man might not have an area of specialty, but he knows, what he does not know. He has a general understanding of general principles; so he knows a little about everything; the *no thing* that runs through it all. Be like Sergeant Shultz on Hogan's Heroes, and know nothing, see nothing, hear nothing and smell nothing.

PERCEPTION

There are a number of different methods of perception, and perceptual awareness: two will be presented, in the attempt to explain awareness without attachment, and perception without concentration (Buddhist meditative view). This will be differentiated from awareness through filtering and/or ignoring non-relevant events and indicators, such as driving a car, through the rain, without windshield wipers.

In the case of the driving in the rain, without wipers, the limited view is transcended by either:
ignoring individual raindrops and/or patterns of rain falling, or
relegating the rain patterns to a low priority.

The driving mentality, has an emphasis on going forward implied, which concentrates on a line type of perception, which is confined primarily to two dimensional, and one direction.

The further limiting of perception ignoring the raindrops, heightens this tunnel vision.

In this environment, not much is considered, perceived or thought: that does not relate to movement and arriving at a destination. Looking through the side windows, is rare, so both sides of a direction are lost. The meaning and reality is totally shaped by it's use for travel by the driver. This is perception limited by attachment.

The non-driving perception of snowflakes can be three or four dimensional, and not limited by direction. One way to see an individual snowflake is becoming conscious of the snowflake pattern, speed of fall, and distance from other snowflakes. Shift the focus to see the composite view of a pattern of many snowflakes falling, or the differences in snowflakes.

One might shift the emphasis of this composite view to:
a) segments of falling snowflakes,
b) movements of groups of snowflakes caused by shifts in the wind, or
c) movements of groups of snowflakes caused by the location of one's eyes
   when viewing, etc.

Consciousness shifting is possible by:
a) being aware of the snowflakes but thinking of something else
   (daydreaming), or
b) seeing a recurring pattern of snowflakes that is common through the
   viewing without concentrating on the individual snowflakes, etc.

With this manner of perceiving snowflakes, there is no limitation or exclusive perception necessary, it is more the manner of focus. One reality is not judged to be better or worse than the other. Multiple realities may simultaneously exist, some would say an infinite number, or that a number of views cease to have a meaning. This is un-attached perception, similar to Buddhist meditation.

MEDITATION BASICS

Meditation might last for a period of 5 - 90 minutes. Before meditation, think of all that has occurred during the day/night, and deal with it then and there, then put it down.

Next think of all that you are going to do, then put it down. The posture for meditation, should be relaxed, centered, balanced and somewhat comfortable, so as not to distract. The two most reliable positions are kneeling, and cross legged.

For the first half of the meditation, inhale and hold the breath, then exhale and hold the breath the same amount of time.

The second half of the meditation, breath naturally.

The first area of meditation, is to meditate on the concept of *no thing*. Not a vacuum, just emptiness without dwelling on any one thing.

In other "religious" news, scientists have discovered that the ancient Buddhist technique of empathetic mediation not only increases neuronalgenesis (more new neurons) but by using magnetic resonance imaging (MRI) they were able to show that this meditative practice can cure obsessive-compulsive disorders (OCD) in the same manner as the drugs that are presently given. Further, this sort of meditation can elevate the natural state of "Happiness" - which has previously been thought of as permanent.

MEDITATIONS

When meditating, do the controlled breathing for 1/2 the time of meditation, then 1/2 the way through, relax and continue your meditation, without controlling your breath and breath naturally.

Meditation might last for a period of 5 - 90 minutes. Before meditating, think of all that has occurred during the day/night, and deal with it then and there, then put it down.

Next think of all that you are going to do, then put it down. The posture for meditation, should be relaxed, centered, balanced and somewhat comfortable, so as not to distract. The two most reliable positions are kneeling, and cross legged.

For the first half of the meditation, inhale and hold the breath, then exhale and hold the breath the same amount of time.

The second half of the meditation, breath naturally.

DIFFERENT MEDITATIONS

Formless Lattice

Generally speaking, it is not usually the best to practice form sets at full speed, full power, or with an intended target. Once a set has been learned at some level; some speed and power are added. After a deeper foundation of the set has been mastered, periodic full speed and power are incorporated, as well as positioning for a possible application.

When a form is practiced without power, speed, analysis, or intended offense/defense; one becomes one with the pure essence of the set, without limiting its use. The move is not defense or offense; yet has components of both. There are none of the attachments of expected results, and is free of the overhead of calculating them. The energy flow and moving meditation aspects are all there is, a much higher plane.

When a particular marital application is not focused on, the move is effectively practiced for all applications.

Similarly, when words are used to explain, demonstrate, or compare a move, there is an extra translation step in the perception, cognition and performance of the move. This translation step; adds and substitutes symbols for essence, cultural experiences, history and the shared lived experiences related to language. This distortion is compounded, when translated to another language.

Although it is better to learn something in the language it was invented in, it is better to use no language at all. Words are not the move, only the container for the idea of the move. Pure imagery is dulled by language. Witness accounts have been shown to be less accurate after they were written.

In mathematics, the area of a curve, can be approximated using steps or blocks to fill up the curve, and calculating the space in the blocks; the more blocks, the more accurate, but it is never equal. Computers use this model. Only calculus differentials will give the true answer of the real curve. In some concepts, the sum is more than the total of the parts.

When a move is followed for what it is, and one becomes one with the move and the sifu as it is executed. This is the highest form of learning; mind to mind. A skill that is thus transferred is colloquially referred to as 'rubbing off on you'. Without this direct transmission, imitation and approximation are all that is possible.

NO THING
The first area of meditation, is to meditate on the concept of *no thing*. Not a vacuum, just emptiness without dwelling on any one thing.

THIRD EYE
Another meditation is to focus on a point before your eyes, and become one with it, not separating the observed point, from the observer (you).

Other good focus points are:
  a) the third eye/upper dan tien area, from a midpoint between the eyes above the eyes, on the forehead to anywhere towards a wall or object (not metal, plastic, electric or glass);
  b) a candle/flame or fire;
  c) a suspended object on a string;
  d) a tree or plant; or
  c) a stone.

ESSENCE of WATER

The next meditation is meditating on the feeling/concept/essence of water except that of wetness. All of your experiences, feelings, and perceptions, and what is common to all of them, the universal. Do not dwell on analytical concepts or theories. Hold feelings and perceptions simultaneously, not as separate aspects, but as different views of the same thing. Qi is most closely associated with this. This is why water is used in some faiths to bless oneself. Holy Water additionally contains some salt, like the water in the human body, and like sea water. Whether you meditate on fresh water, or the concept of sea water, is up to you.

KNIFE PASSING

Another meditation is that of a knife passing through water. Although the knife can cut, the water conforms and yields to the knife. The knife slides through the water, without damage to the water, because the water does not resist, and has no attachments to the water. When this is mastered, along with the *no thing*, distractions are recognized for what they are, and pass through your mind, without reaction.

WALL GAZING

Da Mo or Bodhidharma spent nine years in meditation, where he used to sit facing the rock wall of a cave that's about a mile from the Shaolin Temple. Thus he won the title "the wall-gazing Brahmin". Some stories say that Da Mo burned a hole into the rock that he was meditating in front of.

Wall-gazing, modern psychologists have found, is a great way to induce alpha in both its upper and lower (and even upper theta) frequency ranges.

The technique, called 'ganzfeld' - a German word which means complete field - alpha waves are generated by staring at a blank, preferably white, bright visual field and holding the eyes steadily upon it. A white-wall fulfills this condition. All that is necessary is that the wall occupy the complete field of vision so that distractions are eliminated.

Sit facing as closely as is necessary to have the wall fill the field of vision at:
  a) a wood wall,
  b) a stone wall,
  c) a brick wall,
  d) a white or light-colored blank wall,
  e) a concrete wall,
  f) a wall with some subtle patterns, different enough that everything
     does not look identical, yet no pattern dominates.

Stare at the wall, observing its texture and color patterns. Be aware of differences and commonalities of the wall, without favor to either. Observe patterns forming in the field of vision. At times you may fix all attention upon them. Other times watch them as you would the water surface of a running river.

Empty your mind of all thoughts. Thoughts will continuously pop into your mind but do not dwell on them. Treat your mind as you would treat a child you are taking for a walk. Whenever your attention starts to get stuck on a thought, it must be gently pulled away. Say to it, "Sorry, but we can't stop now, we will think about it another time".

Use peripheral vision, being aware of the focus of your attention
AND the rest of the wall.

One can have a number of focuses when doing wall gazing: a point on the wall, eyes closed, a distance between meditator and the wall and the peripheral vision.

There is quite a bit of discussion about the level, type and benefits of wall gazing, compared to other Buddhist meditations. Some claim it is an advanced method, others have questions. My recommendation is to practice it after the *no thing* meditation.

Wall Gazing is an excellent training method for keeping your awareness and calm, in stressed and distracting situations. It is better than a poker face, since one is not hardened, but aware.

After these have been mastered, the Chi Sau meditation/exercises start.

BUDDHIST MARTIAL CONCEPTS

A martial manifestation of the Middle Way, could be when one practices a move/block, not to concentrate on it being a block or an attack.

For example, when one is walking in the snow, the depth that one's step sinks, is not predictable:

Walking in the Snow
  a) the step could stay on top of hard packed snow, or ice,
  b) one could sink to snow depth, or
  c) the step could sink to knee depth or greater.

One should not attach themselves to expecting one depth, or even that the ankle position or bending; will be the same. The angle of the foot after the fall, relative to the supporting plane, could be pointing:
  a) uphill/ lifted up
  b) level/ prone or
  c) downhill/ tilted down.

One should not attach themselves to how to hold the foot, since one's point of contact might optimally be:
  a) the heel for leaning backwards to prevent forward slide,
  b) the flat of the foot for less sinking or
  c) the ball of the foot for sinking deeply into the snow.

Since the step is dynamic, it is better not to concentrate on form, or a pre-set way of walking. Every step is different. One should not just see with their mind or eyes, but with their feet, and center. The move becomes part of the seeing, not just a result of it!

One should use their arms, in a similar manner, not committing to form, or distance.

A other example; is running in the dark, on a dirt trail, or on the forest floor. If you were to watch and calculate each individual step, the speed would never be greater than a walk.

Letting your foot feel the surface of the ground, and adjusting accordingly, is to run, without a pre-set form.

If one were to think of position, it is ideal to position one's energy and move at half the distance since:
  a) blocking at full distance commits one to the move;
  b) blocking without full extension gives room for:
  c) changing direction,
  d) stopping the move,
  e) responding to another move, or
  f) changing to offense.

A Buddhist meditative concept of practice, would be to not concentrate on the practical application of the move to offense or defense, but to become one with the flow and energy. The move being more than it's use to the practitioner.

A posture that focuses on one's own energy flow, and the feeling of another's Chi through one's center or hand contact, would be more universal and whole. Contrast this to responding, via cause and effect to another's move, which is based on reactions, and have specific limited paths. Better to be there before the move, seeing the Yi and Chi.

In a fighting situation, movements should not be committed to, but should be dynamic and perceptive. Sometimes non-movement is the better than the response. Feints are useless on this level. For the attacker, a feint is not truly dynamic, since it should have the capability to become a full powered blow, depending on the state of the opponent.

When gazing at a candle, there are other angles to be seen, than from the position of the viewer. There are also many things that are missed by the eyes limited of what is around the burning part of the wick, the most obvious being the heat above the flame, and the onion effect of the areas around the center of the flame. Similarly, there is more to the candle, than how we use the candle, or how it directly influences us. Modern physics is starting to see the geomagnetic properties of the flame as well.

There is more to the moon than what we see. The classic example is the Dark Side of the Moon, that we never see, yet is part of the whole moon.

Perhaps the energy around life, is similar to the halo around a candle, some would say this is the aura.

There is more to the whole than the sum of the parts.

Doing Push Hands slowly, non-competitively, and blindfolded: will help sensitize one to these energies, as well as meditation and Chi Sao drills.

JET LI

Jet Li, has an article in the November 2004, issue of Inside Kung Fu, Straight From The Heart, (pages 48, 49 & 72), will shed a light.

"IKF: What brought you to Buddhism?
JL: Buddhism has helped me to find the answers for myself. With Buddhism you look inside yourself for the answer.
...
Martial arts have external and internal training or physical training or mind training. Physical training can help your circulation, or you can meditate or do tai chi and to improve your whole body.
...
There is no philosophy: it is not until you study Buddhism that you will know there is no philosophy, nothing. Because when you believe something you will then find someone will defend themselves against your beliefs. Once you have a point, then another will have their point and the conflict begins. It is better to have no point. That is what we try to do as Buddhists, have no point.
...
Buddhism tells you about the universe and many other things and then you choose which way to go. "

EXERCISE

Before the times of the automobile, most people walked to get around. This developed their legs, stamina and connection to the earth (root); through everyday living. Water had to be carried, wood had to be chopped, and goods packed. Household items had to be made, and all tools were manual, with the user supplying the power.

Most occupations were not white collar jobs, such as being tied to a desk, being a pencil pusher, technician, using a computer, or the telephone. The everyday labor consisted of a large amount of physical work: some strenuous, but most all long and enduring.

With this background most that trained in Martial Arts, did not need the physical workouts at the school where they trained, since they already had it incorporated in their everyday life. These days, there are not many with the same abilities, except those that will train themselves, at times, for 3-8 hour sessions 3-5 times a week, in addition to their daily routine. Most of these trainers, also do other forms of exercise or meditation.

Huo Yuan Chia, Founder of Jing Mo Association sold firewood to make a living, and in 1896 worked as a porter in the Tianjin Huaiqing pharmacy, where he learned more about the world.

Sun Lu Tang was made to run after his teacher's horse to make himself more fit and capable of enduring the training.

STRETCHING

Start with exercises that stretch the limbs to their maximum, slowly, for a count of 10 to 100. This improves form, and the ability to keep the form fully extended, and as close to the ground as for maximum rooting. This is followed with swinging limb exercises; that stretch for moments at the end of the swing.

Workouts should start with repetitions with an emphasis on energy and form; warm up gradually before going full speed to minimize shock related injuries.

This might not be the best for those that do not do a lot of strenuous external physical activity, and whose other primary exercise is like yoga. One can hike a lot uphill, and sometimes carry a pack of 50-100% of their body weight. Do heavy weight lifting, and nunchakus, or rope pulling in fishing. Do not perform these exercises just before training, without these stretches, or your kicks are not effective at much higher than waste level, and arm forms are not fully extended without strain.

If you are going right into push hands, sparring, or weight lifting, best to do only stretch lightly for a few seconds, only a few repetitions, just minutes before.

If one does other training in hiking, climbing, skiing, and mountain climbing, ligaments and tendons are extremely strong. Ski in old style leather boots, not the externally supported fiberglass-shelled modern ones. I have made it to the top of the 14,000 foot peak Mount Shasta, in tennis shoes. This reflects the old school philosophy; that you should strengthen, and rely on your own body, rather than rely on external support and machinations.

This might not be for everyone, but it is great for strengthening the connective tissues, that are critical to dynamic structural changes that must be flexible and adaptive. Internal Martial Arts forms also strengthen this connective tissue of tendons, ligaments, joints and sinews.

When doing a workout at full martial speed, minimize the stretching, to prevent hyper-extension, strains and sprains.

For posture or back problems, do stationary stretches, such as splits, or lotus position, with meditation, or an added secondary stretch.

When doing an internal workout such as Tai Chi, Hsing-i, or Ba Gua, do the Qi Gong stretches with breathing. This distinguishes these from other Qi Gong (Chi Kung); that are moving in smaller circles, or involving internal orbits that circulated energy in the body's center.

After a workout, one might or might not stretch. Some workouts develop a tone, that you do not want stretched, or it will become flaccid. Other workouts develop an energy that is a foundation, or springboard for another activity.

If the workout is long, with many repetitions, or has involved extreme power, do stretching with few repetitions, and a short duration.

CIRCLE STRETCHES

Men will start the circles in a clockwise direction; women counterclockwise. Do 4 -20 repetitions in one direction, and the same number the other way. If bones or ligaments pop, that is OK, but make sure that this does not happen in the same location at the same time in the circle. Inhale as the circle moves toward the body, exhale as the swing goes away from the body.

Popping of joints and ligaments, realigns the body position, releases pressure, and returns the point to a more flexible condition. If this was done correctly, it should not happen again, and repeated popping could be grinding of the joint or an injury.

GRAVITY CIRCLE SETS

Start from the ground with the toes, and work their way up to the head. This insures proper rooting, and structural alignment relative to gravity and the spine. These circles are usually done standing up, but can be done in other supported positions, such as while sitting down.

a) Toe Circles start by placing the ball of the foot or tip of the big toe on the ground, and then revolving the foot and attached leg, around the stationary point on the floor. Energy benefits are added when you add the sway of the knees for momentum that carries the rest of the body with the swing of the circle. This action aids the wave flow from the ground root. This should be done evenly, since the circle is short. It is not always easy to practice coordinating the breathing with a short circle; main thing is to be relaxed.

b) Knee circles can be performed standing erect, or with the hands on the kneecaps, massaging them. By raising the body on the inhale, and lowering on the exhale, one can tone the energy connection to the ground and structural support of the legs.

Another version of the knee circle; is to lean on the right sides of the feet, on the exhale, sinking as the knees angle to the right (right foot's outer knife edge and left foots insole"). At inhale; rise evenly vertical to the center. Next exhale; lean on the left sides of the feet, leaning the knees to the left. This is also used as a downhill skiing exercise.

c) Waist circles can be done with the arms hanging, or with the hands on the back of the hips to massage the kidneys. Make sure to extend the circle fully as it goes in back of your body, as you stretch backward. Try to do this as much as the forward stretch. Wide-stanced circles best for stretching, smaller circles with feet close together better for resetting hip joint and connective tissues.

d) Upper body circles should go backward and downward, as well as forward and downward, emphasize the bending of the back and flow with the arms, along with the back and waist's motion. Circle is long for stretching, shorter for internal movements.

e) Upper torso circles are done with the hand palms over the back of the neck, with the elbows leading the circle.

f) Head/neck circles should be done evenly, since the circle is short. Main thing is to be relaxed.

LEG CIRCLES

a) Should start from the knee, one leg standing, and the other lower leg revolving around the knee as it hangs. After initial circles, inward circle can be changed to a roundhouse kick, the inward to outward circle can be changed to a repetitive side-kick.

b) Full leg circles from the hip in front.

c) Full leg circles from the hip from the side..

FULL ARM WIDE CIRCLES

a) Should start with the shoulders, one way, opposite direction and then alternating.

b) Start the full arm circles; one way, opposite direction and then alternating; full arm figure eights, one way, then the opposite direction.

Internal energy and shoulder strengthening full arm circles using **Unbendable Arm** (page 51) attached to the lower Dan Tien, raising the body on the inhale, as the circle-swing comes toward the body, and lowering it on the exhale as the circle-swing orbits away from the body.

Circles will start with a short, arm radius circle, gradually become larger circles, and then become nearly fully extended; keeping the flexibility of rattan. Do a number of circles in one direction, then the other direction for the same number.

i)   arms held outward to the side away from the body;

ii)   arms held in front, eventually overlapping the circles, yet not contacting;

iii) arms raised toward the sky, but bent more to insure that the upper circle of the hand is at the same height, body will rock back and forth more than up and down;

iv) arms at side, only small circles possible; try and use Lower Dan Tien and body swing only, rather shoulder muscles, since this is easiest done closest to the center.

a) Forearm circles rotating from the elbows; one way, opposite direction and then alternating;
forearm figure eights, one way, then the opposite direction.

b) Wrist circles, one way, opposite direction and then alternating

After loosening first, motion can be used for continuous and returning blocks or strikes.

WRIST STRETCHES

Will loosen wrists, increase Qi circulation, quicken the forearms, prevent injury, and make it harder to for opponents to use Chin Na wrist locks and throws on you, and give you practice to use Chin Na on yourself.

i)   Chin Na # 3

Hold the hands palms vertically together palms facing each other, at solar plexus level with fingers pointed up.

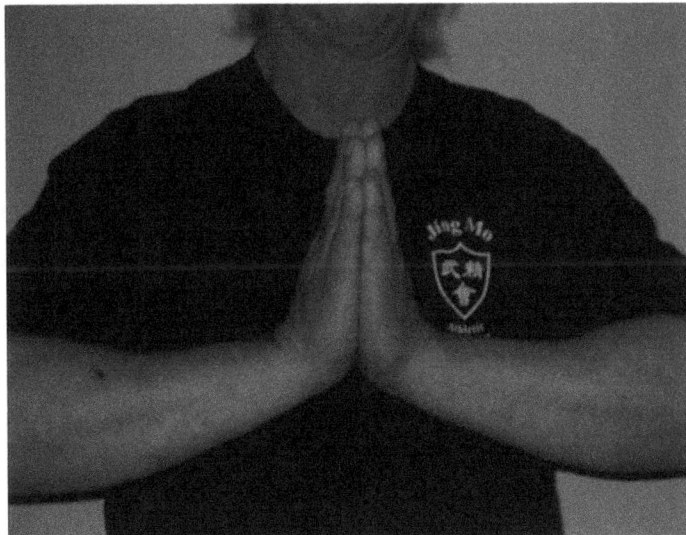

Raise one palm to where the fingers start and
bend the hand backward toward the elbow,
keep forearms horizontally level with the floor.

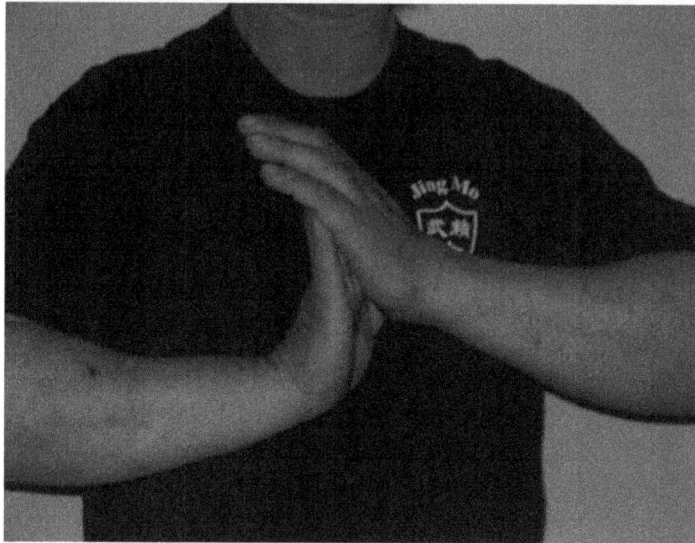

This back and upward move stretches the palm, inside wrist
and inside of the forearm.

ii)　　Put one hand horizontally palm down, thumb inward,
out from the solar plexus,
with the other palm downward hand, hand reach over the
hand, grabbing between the wrist and knuckle.

Inhale as you raise the held lower hand,
bending downward it by the wrist then

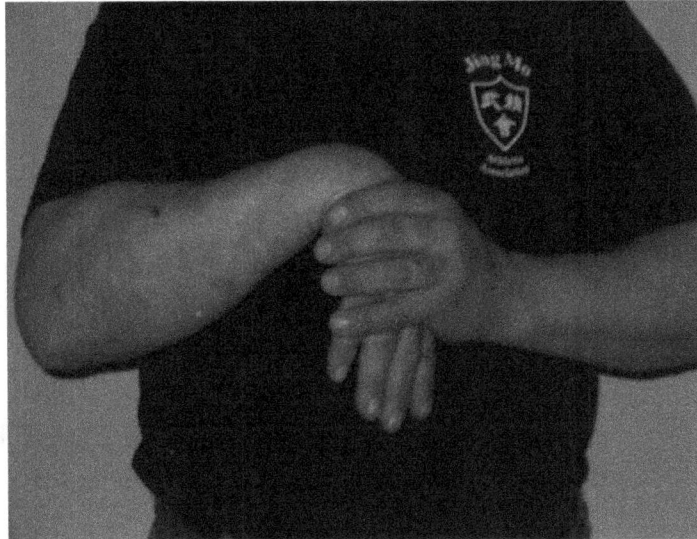

iii)　　Chin Na #7

Hold one hand palm toward you, fingers pointed up;
with the thumb to the outside, at eye level.

Take the other hand, palm facing you and put it past the first
hand and over the first hand with the thumb of the second
hand beneath the knuckle between the ring finger and little
finger of the first hand wrapping the four fingers around the
rest of the hand, capturing the outside of the thumb.

Rotate the first hand' (closest to you) little finger side
toward you by pressing the knuckle point on the hand
causing it to rotate toward you then outward.

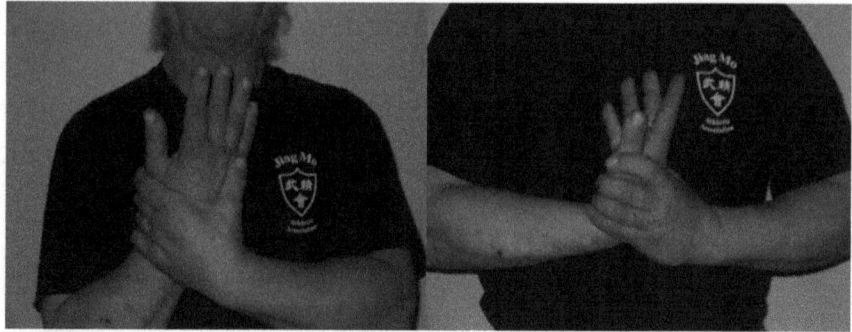

As you rotate, lower the hand combination straight down vertically from eye level to solar plexus level exhaling (this downward rotating motion is like wrapping your hand on a vertical pole and sliding it down as it turns).

Inhale as you raise the hand combination on the same vertical path upward, reversing the rotation so that it returns to eye level with palms facing you.

Inside to outside twist strengthens the back of the hand near the little and ring fingers.

iv)   Chin Na #8, #10

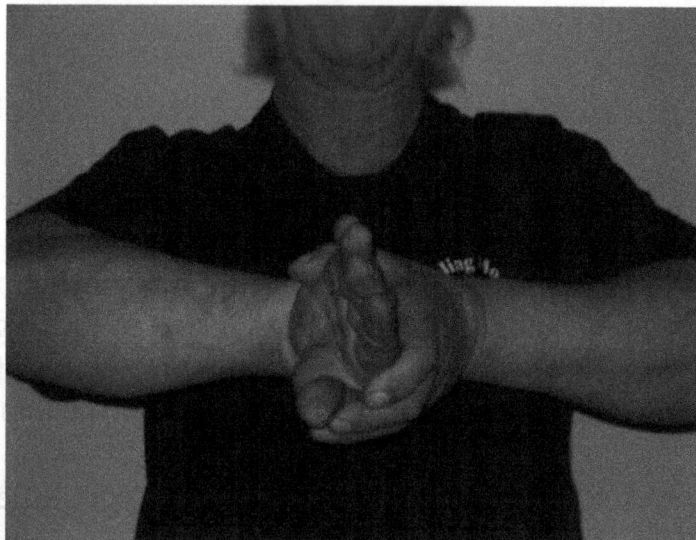

Hold the first hand palm outward you at arms length at solar plexus level, fingers pointed straight out away from you, thumb pointed down so that hand is held sidewise vertically inverted.

Place the second hand's palm flush against the first hand's back with the second hands thumb up, capturing the little finger's ridge hand with the thumb, and the fingers of the second hand wrapping around and capturing the thumb of the first hand above the wrist.

Move the hand pair to the middle of the body at solar plexus level, at arms length.

Inhale as you pull your hands evenly inward toward the solar plexus as the second hand rotates the captured first hand fingertips upward till they are vertical.

Exhale as you drop the captured hand pair, so the captured outward hand is horizontal and fingertips are pointed away from the body and push them horizontally away from the solar plexus to arms length

Outside ridge hand wrist joint is exercised, as well as back of the hand near the index finger with this.

v)   Put one palm outward hand in front of your nose, fingertips pointing horizontally inward, thumb down, with the bent elbow outward.

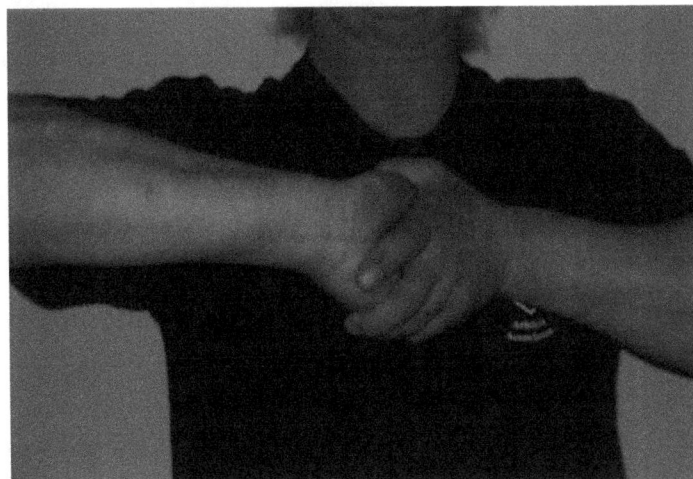

Reach over and past your first hand, with your second hand, palm inward; thumb on top reaching downward over the back of the hand near the little finger, between the wrist and the base knuckle;
fingers capturing the back of the hand near the thumb downward and upward below the wrist.
Rotate the hand pair inward and upward, as you press the hand backward toward the elbow.

You will exercise outside forearm, outer wrist as well as the back of the hand at little finger outside ridge with this palm outward fingers tips inward and downward

vi)   Put one arm at full length, hand palm upward with fingertips pointing away form the body, thumb out ward, arm angling downward to waist level.

With your second palm downward hand reach over the top of the first hand, with your fingers capturing the back of the hand between the thumb and the bottom of the index finger;

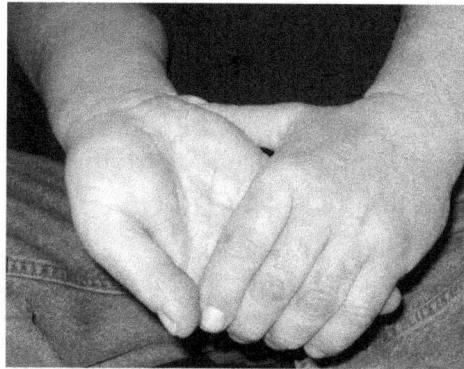

the thumb reaches over the back of the little finger part of the ridge hand between the wrist and the little finger's base knuckle.

Use the second, uppermost hand to push the first hand backward and inward.

This palm out, down, backward to inside stretches the palm, inside wrist and the inside of the forearm.   Entire back of the hand is exercised with this back and downward stretch.

Thumb Stretches

    i)   Done with palm inward hand near the solar plexus with
          thumb straight vertically up:
           backward, toward the elbow;

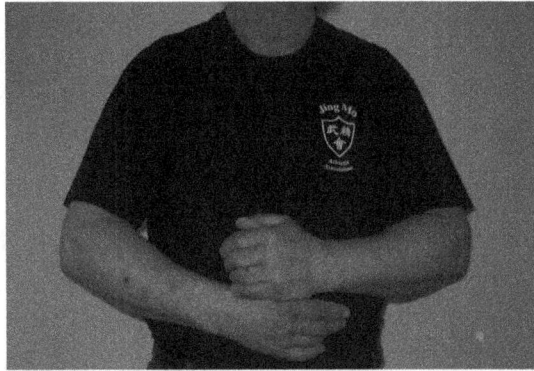

    ii)   Circle the thumb at base joint, clockwise then counter-
          clockwise; outward away from the body;

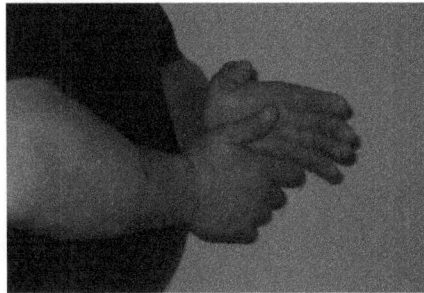

    iii)   Inward toward the body.

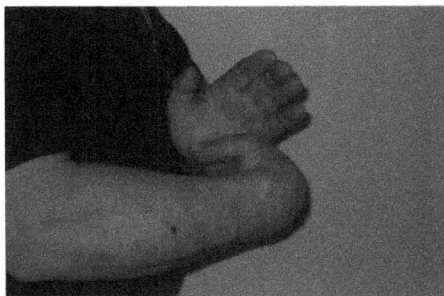

RESET WRIST

Start with palms up.

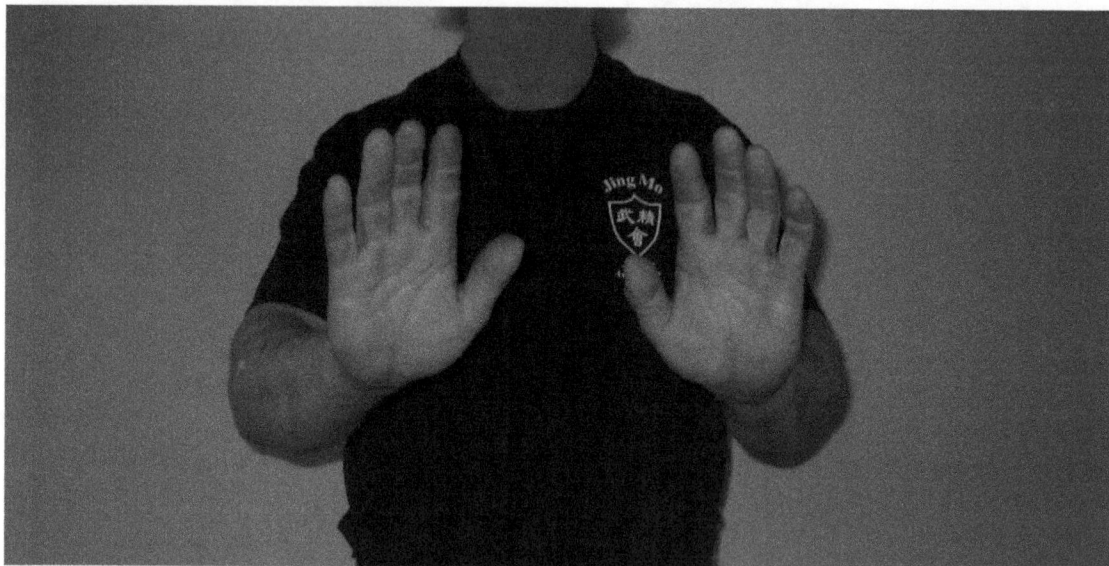

Rotate wrists to the outside and downward.

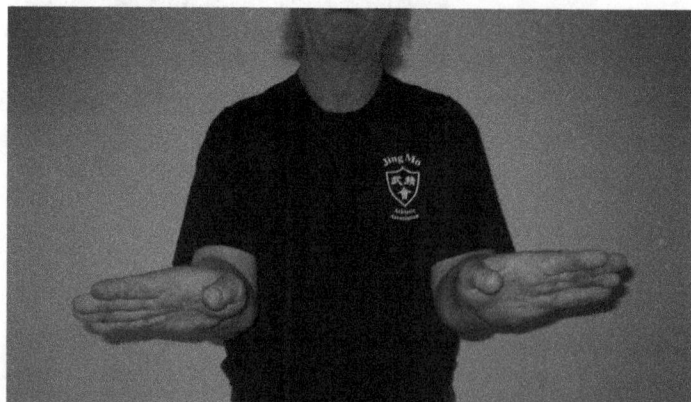

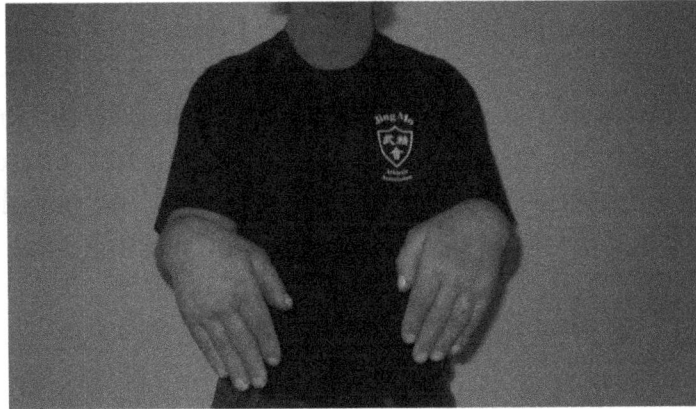

After reaching the bottom; rotate hands upward and inward.

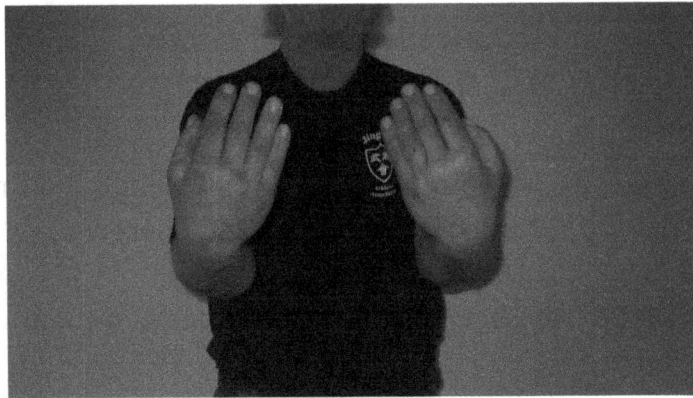

With fingertips pointing up, rotate the hands outward.

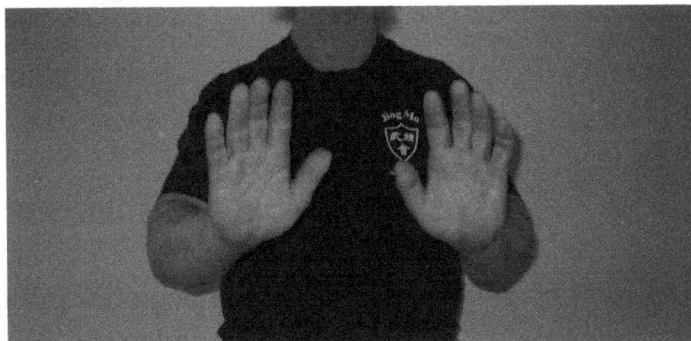

Do four times, reverse direction, do four times, and then reverse to original direction once.

USE YOUR KNEES

In downhill skiing and ice skating, the flow of the foot to the knees is critical in steering and in rooting: try it, perhaps you will not find any difference. This method is taught as a classic principle for vadel and parallel skiing. Use this same method for the solid ground, and for being on a boat (sea legs).

The elbows harmonize with the knees.

One could say that injury and stress could be prevented in lifting and strenuous exercise, by wearing a corset, since it prevents hernia and back injuries. Some use the same logic to minimize knee movement that will minimize stress at the expense of control and power.

HSING-I WORKOUT

Training in forms can give a contuity of thought through their move sequences; introducing patterns, perspectives and energies.

When learning a form from a teacher in person, one can focus on doing the move(s):
1) initially as they last saw it, and wait for the next move to be shown;
2) start with what they last remember about the move and
   fill the rest in with copying the teacher's move;
3) follow the instructor's movement;
4) mirror the teacher's every move as they watch for signs of approval
   or disapproval;
5) do the form set after preliminary ability in the set, in tandem with the
    teacher;
6) both student and teacher in time,
   but not tied to each other by expectations or forced adjustments.

When a form is learned in copy mode alone, one becomes good at following, not going through the changes in their form with independent adjustments, and calculations; does not train the mind to adapt. This adaptation is part of the benefits of the form.

When copied only, one is little more than a robot that has learned another instruction. Sometimes an intelligent person gets good at following by copying, and will display an even flow, tempo and continuity of moves; yet be no better martially, than a choreographed ballerina.

Copying works fine for: acting, tournaments, cocktail conversations and for health. If one wants to learn an internal martial move, it must come from within, to be truly internal since copying by definition is a concept or image brought by another's example.

To polish a picture image, one can go ahead and concentrate on how they appear. Externally, they will look good.

For a deeper understanding, as one goes through a form;
1) one will see with their feet as they walk,
2) bring harmonics into the rhythm of grouped moves,
3) sometimes practice the form with an imagined opponent,
4) concentrate on the power of the moves,
5) focus on the quickness of individual moves,
6) keep similar sequences quick, and pause between them,
7) do the entire form fast,
8) concentrate on the rooting and flow between the moves, and
9) see with your own center of Qi, as it shifts between moves and distance.

Added insight and depth can be attained by doing forms:
1) in dim lit settings and progressing to total darkness or blindfold,
2) in waist deep water,
3) in chest deep water,
4) on uneven surfaces,
5) on a floating surface such as a boat or a dock.

Training to learn new forms with a new focus; can start out as a minor quantitative change on every learned form and then periodically jump qualitatively.

Although forms are an important component of training, no one who has a developed a high level of martial arts through forms alone.

Why be a good actor mimicking an athlete, when you can train as the athlete themselves? Focus on the essence of a move, rather than a copy of that essence.

Better not to rely on any teacher's image, until after you get the basic structure of a set. When one copies a document with a signature or a photo, something is lost that might not be apparent until that copy in turn is copied. What is left is faded, and with less resolution.

When an image is copied, it is a perception of it; not it, nor its essence. After attaining a comfortable level of familiarity of a move, concentrate on doing it correctly for you. Not fast, or powerful; but precisely, or the mistakes are magnified. Power will come next.

There are, in general, three branches of Hsing-i: Shang, Hopei and Honan. Sun Lu Tang learned Hopei Hsing-i and later evolved his Hsing-i into his own sub branch of Hopei.

=========

FACING NORTH

Form practice starts facing north, to orient oneself, inside and out, day or night.

In a bow, through sinking; one can connect back to the ground.
Through raising; one can bring energy up through the ground.

Much of it relates to the grounding to the earth's center of geo-magnetic energy and gravitational forces.

Expansion and inhalation can draw in the sky's/heaven's energy.
Exhalation can release power, impurities, and bad energies.

Some animals and people are sensitive to Magnetic North. It has been discovered that some have magnetite in their Pineal Gland (near Upper Dan Tien and Third Eye).

Birds are documented finding their way north through this.

Properly trained, people likewise can find north by feel.

Being sensitive to geo-magnetics, affect your rooting, hence your bow.

When one's sense of direction is based on True or Magnetic North:
it works at an location,
in almost all geographical formations, (as good as a compass),
in the dark or day,
inside or out,
whether your blind or deaf,
in any country, and in any language.

A bow can be a physical and spiritual connection/relationship to Earth Qi.

Some also theorize the origin of 7-Star Mantis;
the Big Dipper = 7 stars.

Additionally, the Solar Flare driven Solar Particles and Aurora Borealis concentrate at the poles.

Magnetic minerals in the earth are primarily iron (ferrous) based. These are highest in concentration at the densest iron core of planets.

This iron core serves to center, the spin and gravity of the revolving planet. This action between two revolving bodies and the ground, is used in the dynamics of two sparring or push-hand partners such as:

1) When one balances a car tire, they are truing the center axis of the
    spinning tire, eliminating wobble in the orbit.
2) A ball that has a much smaller weight put on it;
    a) when weighted in the center can go farther (depending on weight)
    b) when weighted on the outside of the ball (circumference),
       the ball will screwball to a shorter distance.
3) Two engaged opponents will spin depending upon their center of chi,
    and the center of chi between them.
4) The physics of impact force is dependant on the centering,
    as well as density distribution of its payload (bullet).
5) One taking or throwing a penetrating strike,
    is affected by one's rooting, center of chi, and resonance with energy
    dispersed.

Many of the rules of planetary gravity apply to two spheres on a frictionless plane. Two iron balls will be pulled to each other, on a smooth level surface.

The effects of the earth on martial power, is considerable, although sometimes subtle.

The geo-magnetic orientation of north is a based upon these properties of earth.

The forms not included are:
Continuous Linking Fist (links elements),
Mix Shape Fist (links elements and animals),
Eight Shape Fist (contains four elements and four animals),
Five Element Fist (Creation),
Mutual Destruction Fist

The Hsing-i forms presented here are:
Twelve Animals
Eagle-Bear (combination set), Dove, Hawk, Chicken, Sparrow, Monkey, Dragon, Horse, Snake, Turtle, and Tiger.
I learned Alligator from Mr. ST Ying, "The Old Man" at the Chinese Baptist Church in Berkeley. He used that in place of Turtle.

Five Elements:
 Metal, Water, Wood, Fire & Earth

Alternatives are presented in the Hsing-i forms:
   1) more applications give a wider range of dynamics,
   2) increases adaptability:
       a) are martial effective,
       b) fosters a wider and more rounded consciousness
           (definition of intelligence is the ability to adapt).

METAL

Energy is passed from rear rising hand, to the forward falling axe hand, as the other rising hand closest to the body overtakes the far hand, propelling it past the previous far hand, as it strikes diagonally downward. As both fists move diagonally upward, before the one fist pasts the other on the way up, they travel a path aligned with the Lower Dan Tien, much like the position and feeling of holding a flag pole in a waist belt doing honor guard.

On the way down, the other hand follows a line from the striking axe hand, to the center of the Lower Dan Tien. This movement is like running your closest hand along the ax handle when chopping wood

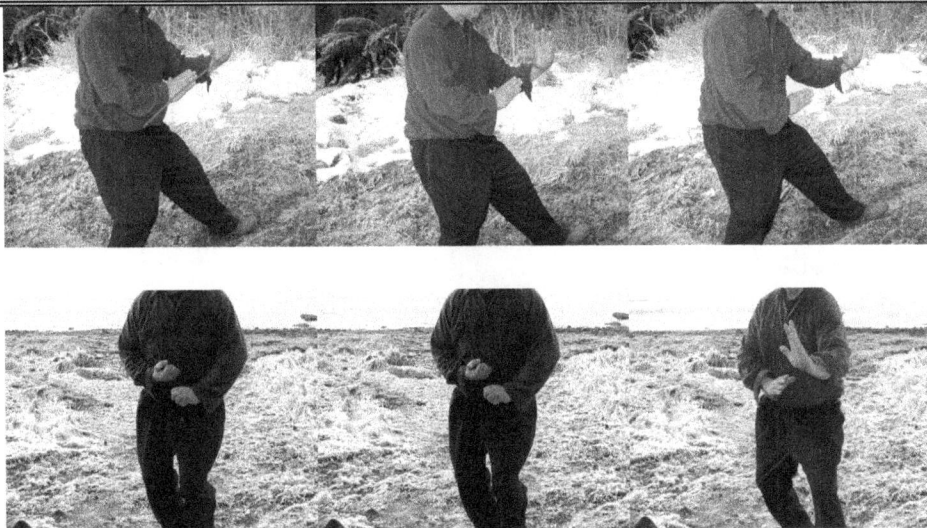

The front left palm, sinks with the front left knee: collecting.
One springs the Water fist upward; carrying the body forward.

Energy is passed forward to the right rear hand as the rear hand advances with the right foot stepping forward even with the left leg.
As the right leg passes the left leg to become the new front leg, this transferred upward energy from the left hand, has already peaked and is now cresting as the downward fall of the downward-splitting right axe-hand.

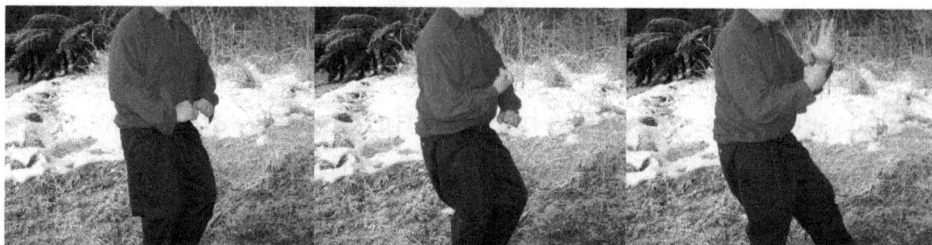

Internal power is gathered by the first rising hand, before it is overtaken by the opposite rising hand (which becomes the far axe hand).

Inhale while drawing the energy in toward the Lower Dan Tien, as the palm downward hand turns down and inward, to a palm upward uppercut. Exhale, expelling it out as you drop; passing it from one hand to the other. This passing can be driven by the step, and drive the step.

When at rest, the rear foot propels the rising; which is then sunk into the far ax hand.

When advancing, the foot steps at the same time the hand is overturned, as it overtakes the other fist.

When the axe hand drops, the elbow moves downward and outward, following the rib cage as the front heal foot is pedaled along the sole toward the toes, driving the front hand through the Lower Dan Tien.

After the foot is flattened then elbow drop stops, continued by the forearm-axe-hand's diagonal drop splitting forward.

Successive forward strikes can be viewed as a horizontal 8-pattern

Best attack pattern when an opponent 's strikes targeting you from navel to solar plexus height.
1) Drilling upper-cut with rear hand acts to block vertically upward with fist
2) After apex of uppercut, front hand reaches upward from behind raised rear hand, and acts as a cross-arm block.
3) Uppercut fist 'throws the ball' into front axe hand, which continues it downward in axe hand, as rear hand 'slides along the axe handle'
   (the line from the Lower Dan Tien focused through:
   first the rear palm then the index finger).

This drawing action of the rear hand is lead back by
the sinking base of the palm of the extended front axe head-fist by
the sinking root of the rear leg, plumbed by the spine.

Martial practice could include:
 1) using the front hand as a grab;
 2) having the front grabbing hand to pull the opponent's arm to:
       a) un-root the opponent,
       b) pull the opponent closer,
       c) pull you closer to the opponent and closing the gap;
 3) using the first rising hand as an uppercut, or upward pushing block.

Related forms are a rising-falling combination is used by Sparrow, and with the reverse hand in Dragon. In Eagle-Bear, the hands are different; but the rising and falling combination is similar, with the steps timed differently.

WATER

The front upper palm hand as it overturns into a downward palm down block; can transfer the energy to the rear upper striking hand, as it overturns, as if pouring into the lower cup holding hand.

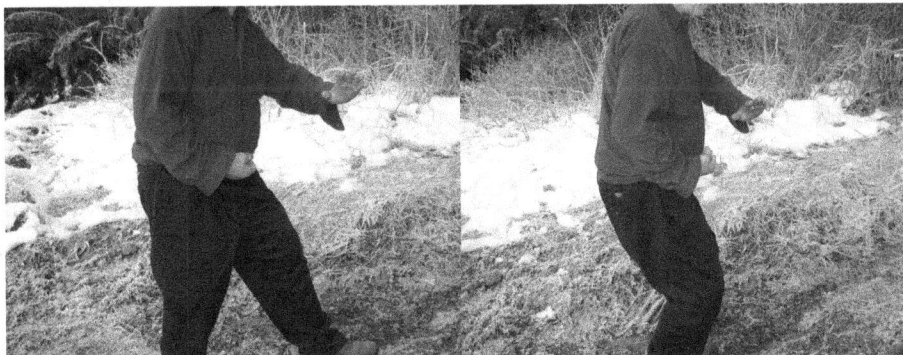

Internal power is gathered by the rear-hand: draw the energy in toward the Lower Dan Tien; as the palm downward-hand turns down and inward to a palm upward uppercut; inhaling. The rear strike will be more rooted, by next pooling this transferred-gathered energy beneath the ground of the rear foot, up to six feet below the surface.

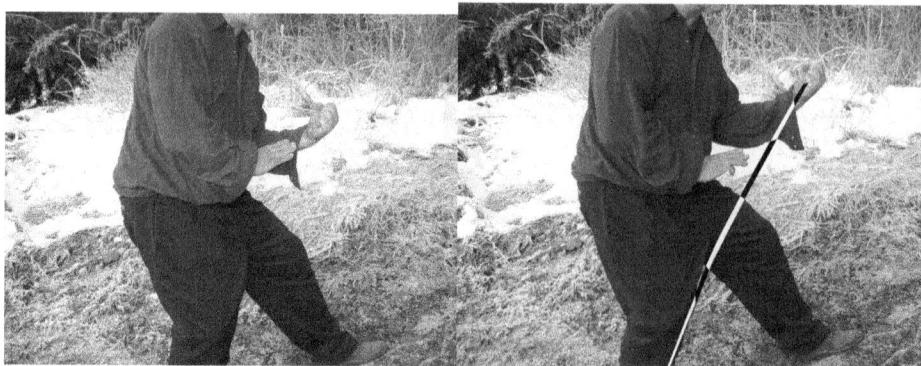

This is the root platform from which the springing rising hand strikes upward in an uppercut; exhaling.

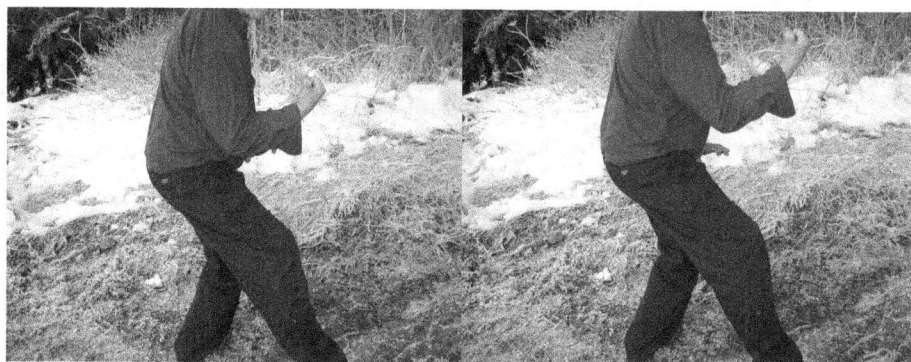

Related forms of Snake, and Alligator also use rising energy, as well as the beginning of Eagle-Bear.

WOOD

The front hand's brush knee type downward block and forward step are propelled with the forward drop; which is controlled by the rear foot and focused with the front foot. Inhale while starting the brushing-knee, gathering or sticking to opponent's strike. Exhale starts at drop, as arms pass midpoint: going forward from the Lower Dan Tien.

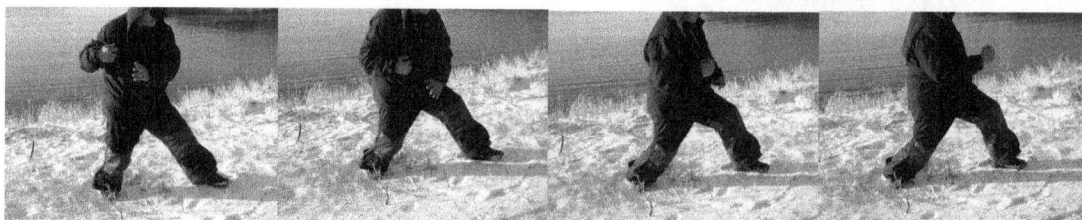

The brush knee and forward foot movement propel the rear reverse punch arrow hand. This can be done either by:

1) the front blocking arm's downward swinging momentum combining with a body sinking, in-place, which combines with the initial swing of the rear hand's reverse punch;

2) the front arm, blocking hand sticks to the contact of the opponent, and followed by the rear hand's reverse punch;

3) the blocking hand grabs what is being blocked, and pulls you forward, with the rear reverse punch;

4) the blocking hand grabs what is being blocked, and pulls your opponent toward you, into your rear reverse punch.

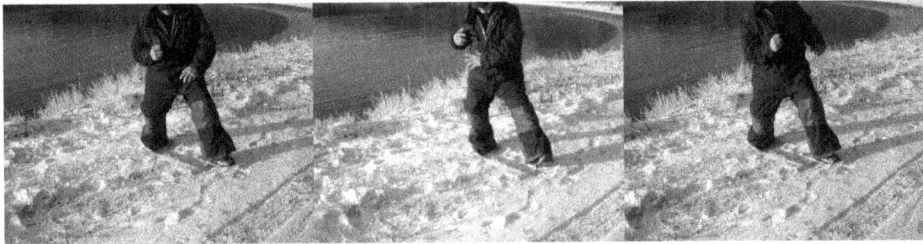

FIRE

The upper blocking front hand can raise the opponent's arm, or be ducked under. Contact of the opponent can be controlled by the front upward blocking hand to:

a) deflect the power of a strike inward,

b) tap-climb inward with the rear striking hand.

c) pulling the opponents arm to:

   i) bring the opponent closer,

   ii) bring you closer to the opponent, closing the gap.

Inhale as you gather both arms; the farthest extended arm then being pushed by both the Lower Dan Tien and rear hand extending.

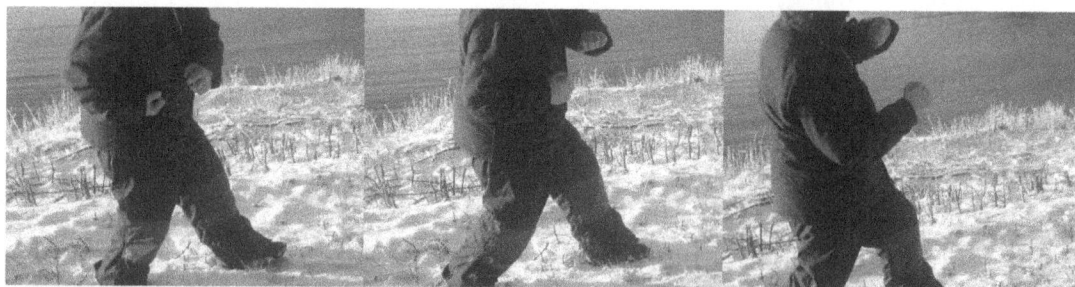

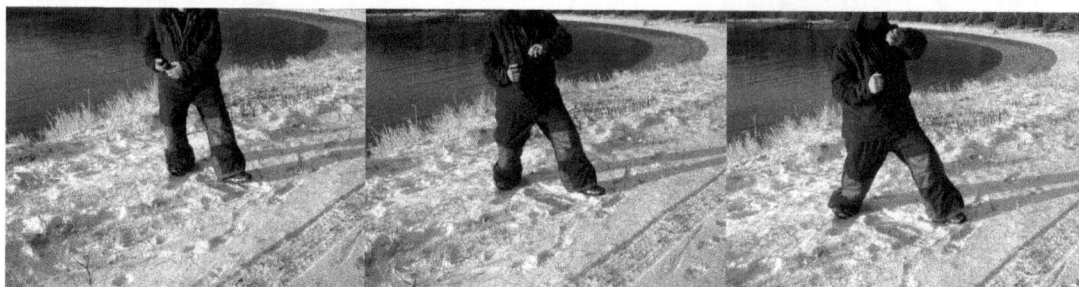

Upper arm blocking fist's upward rotation, unfolds the lower arm's reverse mid to high front punch, as it could potentially roll under the attacker's incoming mid to high punch.

One arm's energy can act to mask, and pave the path of the next arm's. One application could be paved paws, one to grab; pulling the opponent into the other arm's blow. An energy concept of forward fist's application, might be similar to a multiple stage rocket (Monkey Jump for the feet).

In Chess this is hiding behind an attack is called 'Check Under Cover'. When one piece is moved, just by it's relocation; clears the path for another piece to attack the opponent. Those skilled in its use, attack with this piece as it simultaneously releases the barrier to the attack path it was blocking; resulting in two attacks with one move.

The first turn on Fire uses two Hsing-i Alligators; that are reeled a little more upward, as in the Tai Chi move 'reeling silk',
left hand in front moving inward to outward,
thumb or ridge hand leading,
started by left advancing step, of former rear left leg;
followed by right handed Alligator.
The second turn, uses only one Alligator; more upward, but not reeled out, as in the Tai Chi move 'reeling silk'.

EARTH

The tearing of cotton is felt near the Lower Dan Tien between the two hands palms; as you exhale.

The action of the two hands in this inner-circle orbit, is as if they were each posts on each side of a revolving disc, on opposite sides of the circle. This feeling is heightened on the turn.

One can also focus on the keeping the two fists like a bolo:
the front palm downward hand being on one side of the orbiting circle,
and the rear palm upward hand, being on the opposite side of the circle, each fist orbit on the same orbit-plane, equidistant; keeping pace with each other.

Tearing cotton focuses on grounding and power,
the bolo orbiting increases the speed and surprise.

The front far hand inhales as it is extended outward and inward; passing the energy to the upper palm of the bottom rear hand.

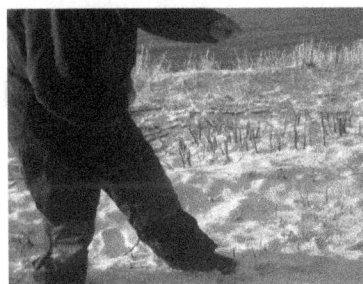

The first strike of front ridge hand from outside to inside; can be preceded by an open palm upward-to-downward inward flip of the wrist,
to sweep an area before the second rear hand strike.

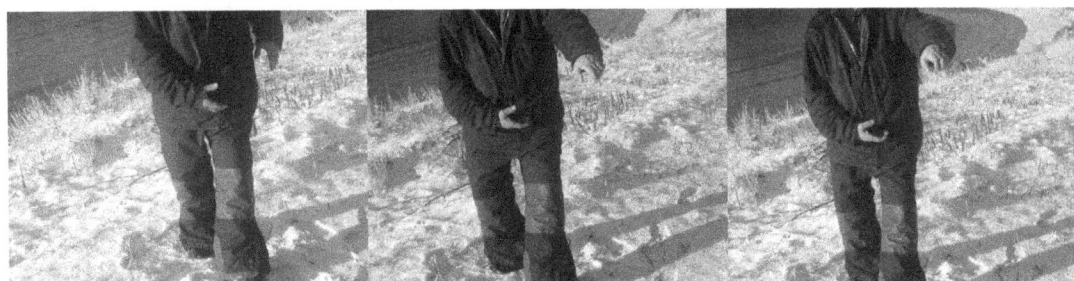

Marital application can include:

  i)   using the upper first farthest extended hand as an
        outward to inward ridge hand strike then using the
        rear hand as an inside to outside block-strike.

  ii)   keep the upper first hand in a continuous palm down **circle**
        with the other second lower hand in the same timed orbit in the
        opposite direction.

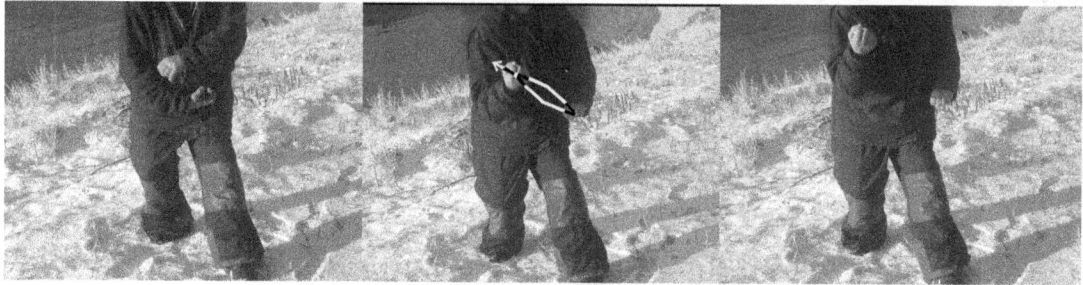

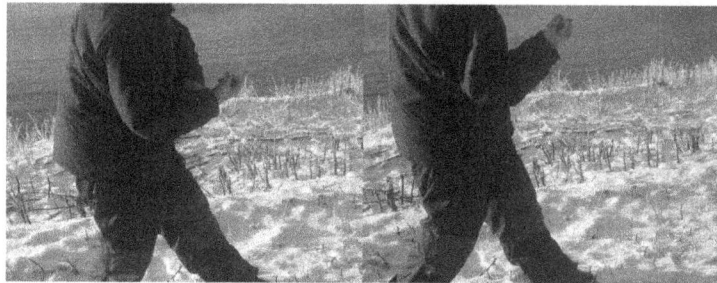

The related form of Horse; uses this with the front hand instead of the rear.

FIVE ELEMENT TRAINING

Start learning the forms first, with the synchronization of the forward step,
as shown above.

Learn the Hsing-i Five Element Spear for whole body movement, timing of
the forward and rearward step; for blow propagation and moving the whole
body forward.

Next, learn the Hsing-i Element Fists with the added rearward step timed
with blow delivery and positional advancing.

FIVE ELEMENT FISTS

Good for martial drills, when responding to a strike. All elements can block with one hand as they strike with the other.

Blocking hand should be sensitive to opponent's strength, momentum, and root. The blocking energy should be the same, whether it pulls you to the opponent, or the opponent toward you. Power of your force is shaped relative to opponent's center of Qi and its relationship to his root and striking target area.

ANIMALS

MONKEY

One of the best for closing the gap, and using longer distances, that are shielded with a continuous flurry of arm movements. Monkey step is used by other Shaolin systems such as Praying Mantis and Drunken Styles.

The far front hand lowers; inhaling while gathering energy from the ground, and then springs up to carry the next move of the far front foot stepping forward. This step forward pulls the Lower Dan Tien; which in turn pushes out the opposite hands forward-striking palm, exhaling, that carries the rear foot and body with it.

Keep a Slinky type or bungee-chord connection between the arms, Lower Dan Tien, legs and the ground.

DRAGON

One can get the longest distance covered with Dragon.

Left hand goes upward in drilling fist, inhaling while bringing with it the right rear leg. The right rear leg is lifted and as it rises it brings the right rising fist. The two fists are aligned vertically and are combined and timed with the rear leg movement in an upward swing; that is carried horizontally by the momentum, at that point like traveling along clothesline pulley.

Both rear and front hands can form a single Hsing-i Water, on the rise, during the leg tuck, but before the kick.

Exhale as you descend: extending the palm downward and/or outward.

After the Double Water Fists, rear tucked leg, kicks out from the Lower Dan Tien; changing the vertical propulsion to horizontal. This propels you along the 'clothes line'.

Time now to spread the force, in an undulated J Dragons falling splitting palm, drawn out and extended by the rear palm downward hand's move . Both hands are moving away from the body's center and away form each other; along the horizontal waist plane.

Dragon undulates with step, with the rising and falling Martial Power of Water and Metal. This does not imply any theory about element theory, or acupuncture, only the physics of the blow.

Different practice distances:

1) Short. The rear leg steps heel first with toe toward the outside, close hand changes to palm down and drops toward the Lower Dan Tien, throwing toward the front hand, which is striking palm downward.

2) Medium. The rear leg heel-kicks the opponent's knee.

3) Long. The rear leg kick carries the body as the hands rise; almost as if they are catching a clothes line pulley in the air, riding it (your leg catapulted energy as it moves like whip through your body).

HORSE

Forward palm downward hand is pulled toward the Lower Dan Tien, as it passes outward, from inside to outside, it is pushed by the rear leg and directed by the Lower Dan Tien, while grabbing and concentrating the fist in an inside to outside block, palm inward. This action can block, or sweep defensively. The front arm inside to outside block can gather energy, inhaling while pulling the rear had to midpoint, exhaling afterward.

The front hand must be dynamic and sensitive to the contact and energy of the opponent;
   1) a rigid and strong opponent's arm is stuck to, then you side step slightly, and used to pull you, and your rear hand front punch forward;
   2) a light and quick opponent's arm is lightly tapped or trapped bending your wrist backward and downward;
   3) in the absence of an opponent's strike, it is used as a sweep, or an inside to outside strike.

The palm upward rear hand is pulled by your front hand, as it reaches the strike's midpoint, where it is turned palm downward, drilling forward through any opponent's countermeasure. This action's momentum carries you, stepping forward, then you ground as you direct the force.

The rear hand can be used from the ground upward; or from high, grounding downward. This must be decided before starting the horse combination; use 1) or 2). In either case the force is started with the leg, but later directed by the Lower Dan Tien.

1) When coming from the ground upward, the rear leg pushes the body at level forward and then pushes the rear hand turned front punch upward.

2) When coming from high down ward, the rear leg is raised as it is moved forward, as one would raise the knee for a kick, propelling the body a good distance forward, before it crashes downward, carrying the power of the rear hand, turned front hand strike.

   a) Traditional: front hand starts with inside outside block, followed by rear leg rising, then advancing to front, carrying the front punch.

b) Crazy Horse, prize fighting aggressive attack:
- i)   Front leg is raised for low jumping font kick which carries body and front punch far forward.
- ii)   Front leg is raised far enough to clear ground in an elongated sliding step, carrying the body and propelling the front punch.

In the downward version of Horse's front punch, one should sink their step. In the upward version of Horse's front punch, a Mantis Springing Step (Bong Po) can be used.

SNAKE

As in Chicken, the first front hand movement, is initiated with the quick, darting front leg, in an empty-sliding-step. Scissor stepping: the feet being the handles of the scissor, the Lower Dan Tien the axis, and the hands the cutting edge; squeezed from the body's moving ground root. The far front hand lowers, blocking palm downward; then gathering energy from the ground, inhaling, being propelled by the rear leg, and then springs up as it extends; continuously or changing to a level forward direction.

The extension is sprung out, exhaling as in Water. The rear leg; urges the squeezed-pedaling of the front font forward. From the opponent's view; Snake comes out of nowhere, so it has the advantage of surprise. The front foot's step forward, can add an inward knee strike angling inward; as the front hand strikes downward and forward. One could also combine the two hand movements (first hand's outside to inside palm side block and second hand's upward forward fist), into a one-handed dynamic block-strike by sensitized contact of the opponents' striking area with the sliding palm side of the forearm.

SPARROW

1) Energy is passed from rear rising hand, to the forward falling axe hand, as the other rising hand closest to the body overtakes the far hand, propelling it past the previous far hand, as it strikes diagonally downward.

As both fists move diagonally upward, before the one fist pasts the other on the way up, they travel a path aligned with the Lower Dan Tien, much like the position and feeling of holding a flag pole in a waist belt doing honor guard.

2) On the way down, the other hand follows a line from the striking axe hand, to the center of the Lower Dan Tien. This movement is like running your closest hand along the ax handle when chopping wood.

3) Internal power is gathered by the first rising hand, before it is overtaken by the opposite rising hand (which becomes the far axe hand). Inhale while drawing the energy in toward the Lower Dan Tien, as the palm down hand turns down and inward, to a palm upward uppercut. Exhale, expelling it out as you drop; passing it from one hand to the other. This passing can be driven by the step, and drive the step.

4) When at rest, the rear foot propels the rising; which is then sunk into the far ax hand.

5) When advancing, the foot steps at the same time the hand is overturned, as it overtakes the other fist.

5) This is done on the same side, rather than alternating sides as in Metal; the rear toe-outward leg shuffles forward propelling the rising fist: this combination propelling the front toe forward leg, in a Slinky (physics toy coil) manner followed by the crashing down of axe-hand.

The action between the first Metal and the second Metal, can be seen as the sparrow's wings coming together before beating downward

Successive forward strikes can be viewed as an inline cascading double axe-hand; repeating 1) through (5.

Martial practice could include:
1) using the front hand as a grab;
2) having the front grabbing hand to pull the opponent's arm to:
    d) un-root the opponent,
    e) pull the opponent closer,
    f) pull you closer to the opponent and closing the gap;
3) using the first rising hand as an uppercut, or upward pushing block.
4) repetitive rising and falling piston action in a flurry of two axe-hand sets, shuttling your steps forward;
   Water dynamic block striking uppercut with the rising fist and then striking one side of the head or collarbone with the falling ax-hand.

In the repetitive double axe hand, the second axe rising/axe hand can remove opponent's block of first axe hand.

TIGER

Hands are held with the tiger mouths facing each other:
  index fingertips angled to be pointing toward each other with a little gap,
  thumbs pointing directly to each other:
  forming a triangle, with the thumbs being the base, and
  the index fingers being the side (hypotenuse) .

Both palm downward fully extended arms, starting at shoulder height; drop their elbows, and are pulled downward and toward your center by your Lower Dan Tien; inhaling, then rise along your chest to solar-plexus level.

As the arms reach your Middle Dan Tien, fingers scoop - pointing downward, then horizontal as they are rising to shoulder height; changing to vertical, as they continue to rise to head level, pointing palm outward.

This scooping action can be used to grab or stick to an opponent's outstretched arms.

While the hands reach your Middle Dan Tien, keep the elbows close to your ribs and lower than the hands.

Depending on force and defensive reaction, the hands continue to rise from shoulder height, to as high as your head. The gap between the hands increases from little at solar plexus height to shoulder width or greater at head level.

The scooping action from waist to solar plexus height, is transformed to rising energy, much like the movement of white crane, without the hand posture. The scooping action, is augmented by drawing the body back with it, which is more pronounced in the feet, which can be raised, as in white crane.

At the arms full height, the backward draw of the foot energy is transferred to the rear leg, which is lifted and catapulted with the step forward. The former front leg becoming the new rear leg.

This down and forward movement of the now front leg; carries the body with it, in the same fashion. This downward body movement is centered and directed by the Lower Dan Tien into the palms, which are facing outward and depending on application of a block or dynamic strike-block; into the ridge hands. The ridge hands can slide along the opponent's striking or outstretched arms, or directly; terminating inside the opponent's chest, or beyond

The fingertips up, palm outward hand pair is directed down and forward to the opponent's chest or collarbone area.

Non-apparent motion is like Water released from on high between the hands, pulled through the Lower Dan Tien from below the ground as an axe hand (Metal), carrying the stance and moving-root with it; directed by the Lower Dan Tien; Yi focusing at midpoint (between hands, Chi -Center relation).

The Slinky or bungi chord type step; is employed after the front leg comes down, to have the rear leg follow the movement forward.

DOVE

Step 1 Start

As in Tiger, apparent motion is started with both arms: they are simultaneously drawn inward as energy is pulled inward, scooping: pooling the water bucket as one inhales into the Lower Dan Tien. Those practicing Shaolin White Crane, benefit from this internal.

As in Tiger, non-apparent motion is started in the ground: directed by the Lower Dan Tien; Yi focusing at midpoint (between hands, Chi -Center relation).

Step2 Midpoint

As in Tiger, centering between mid arms, mid stance and Lower Dan Tien

Step 3 Ending

As in Tiger, apparent motion is issued by both arms: they are simultaneously pushed forward at level, or upward: springing the gathered Chi through both arms, like water through two pipes, to crest through the fists into the opponent, as one exhales from the Lower Dan Tien.

Non-apparent motion is like Water pushed from the ground, carrying the stance and moving-root with it; directed by the Lower Dan Tien; Yi focusing at midpoint (between hands, Chi -Center relation).

Dove can be adjusted to either
1) pull yourself to the opponent or
2) pull the opponent toward you;
and then delivering the uppercut, the energy is the same, see Forearm Throw (page 66).

CHICKEN

Start with San Ti stance, left foot forward. Left foot is empty.
Left front hand retreats toward the body downward, in a downward palm block; palm downward, fingertips pointing forward away from the body.

As you are blocking downward, you sink into the rear leg, slightly crouching. This builds the platform from which you launch a flurry of three spear hand strikes.

Initial first front step is initiated in a Ba Gua (Pa Kua) Snake Step or Ba Gua Chicken Step; propelling the first front hand movement; quick, darting spear hand, palm downward and level. Shaolin Snake benefits from this tandem motion of hand and legs.

First left spear hand is accompanied with the empty sliding short step of the left foot. This is followed with the right foot pushing off the ground from the ball of the foot; transferring energy through the Lower Dan Tien to the right rear spear hand. As the right rear hand is propelled forward, the right rear leg un-weights, sliding up even with the left foot in a short step. Both feet are together, at this point, knees slightly bent.

Third left spear hand is done as the first, with the left foot going in front.

The flurry of spear hands cascade on one another; the hand motion of the two, looking similar to the pedals on a bicycle. This pattern is continuous and can block any of the opponent's countermeasures.

If the opponent throws a low punch, dynamic block-strike downward, on top of the opponent's arm, and slide along top of their arm with the spear hand.

One can use the upper base of the end of the arm, as a Mantis or Crane upward block: wrist bent with fingertips downward The dynamic block-strike used against a high punch, is directed underneath the opponent's arm, and slides underneath their arm to the armpits, chest, or head areas.

This is a rapid fire flurry of attacks.

HAWK

Step1
Left foot is in front, in San Ti stance.

Rear right foot steps up even, and sends the rear right driving/sinking hard fist to root in the ground, reinforced downward; hand looping in an arc up to head level, at its apex, and the as it falls down to shoulder level; it is reinforced by the rear stationary left hand, which acts like a rocket tube. Action is like lead sap bag punched through tube ground-ward.
This movement is and upside down vertical J-pattern.
One can 'nail' this strike to the ground, and their advancing rear step.

Step2
The left hand is drawn toward the Upper Dan Tien, then sunk to the Lower Dan Tien, and then shot downward and forward, as the front foot slides forward, into a bow stance.

This is a lowering horizontal J-patterned front punch at targets abdominal height or lower. This movement is an upside down version of Hsing-i Snake.

Connection from striking hand to Lower Dan Tien is like Saltwater Taffy.

This is a splitting axe hand:
  comes from high vertical, and is drawn forward horizontally,
  by the heel rocking stomp,
  propagated from the root of rear foot and
  directed through the Lower Dan Tien connection of the front leg;
  with a stomp.

J-pattern is a horizontal J, with the curved side up;
this pattern is horizontally opposite to Hsing-i Snake.
Snake patter is also a horizontal J, but with the curved side down.

In both Snake and Hawk, power is accumulated and launched in the short curved area of the J. Snake s rising, so closer to Hsing-i Water, whereas Hawk is falling, as in axe hand.
Step3 Option A Folding Collapsing Elbow
   a) Right foot steps forward, surpassing left foot, to become the new front foot;
   b) right heel drives the right fist Water (uppercut),
      and the right elbow vertically upward; as the

130

c) left hand grabs right fist, using forearm leverage directed by Lower Dan Tien.

Step3 Option B Folding Collapsing Elbow (not in form set)
   d) Right foot steps forward, even with left foot;
   e) right heel drives left elbow vertically upward as
   f) right hand grabs left fist, using forearm leverage directed by Lower Dan Tien.

180 degree turn has energy passed overhead to a reverse down ward splitting fist.

EAGLE-BEAR

Step1 Bear Rising
As in Hsing-i Water that is more vertically accentuated

Step2 Midpoint Transfer
Similar transfer of energy, from rising to falling; as in Hsing-i Metal

Step3 Eagle Diving
As in Dragon; forward and/or downward; with either a downward facing palm, full eagle claw, or using the thumb for a point strike.
Can be developed into an Internal Iron Palm Strike.

TURTLE

The bottom palm upward hand, is held near it's side next to the Lower Dan Tien inhaling while gathering Qi. The forward front hand starts palm upward., on top of the other hand with a gap, at midline of the Lower Dan Tien. Both hands slightly swing with the ball of Qi on top; the forward hand leading and pivoting at the index finger.

The swing is started with the rear foot, as it gains momentum and goes forward, it is directed by the Lower Dan Tien, exhaling; carrying the body forward. When near completion one sinks, to propel the front hand as it turns upward and forward, striking with the ridge hand.

131

Since Turtle does not have bone based linear movement, it is one of the best for developing internal striking energy, which eventually can be directed without the need of limb or skeletal movement.

The Spear as a Teacher
Hsing-i Five Element Spear

In many martial arts systems, weapons are only taught to advanced students. One exception to his was in the early 1970s I studied Aikido, from a school that emphasized ki (chi), currently most do not. The short staff was used to show how to move the body as a unit and use this to throw people. Skill in the staff was not encouraged, only its use as a teaching tool of empty hand.

Hsing I Five Element Spear is well suited to be taught to beginning and intermediate students, after or as they study the empty hand Hsing I Five elements. Hsing-i empty hand was based on the principles of the previously developed Five Element Spear.

In older times, students were more familiar with Chi, meditation, and intrinsic power. Students stayed with schools for longer.

In modern times, many will come with backgrounds in sports or karate, and have previous training that must be overcome.

The teaching axiom of going from the known, to the related unknown, can have unintended consequences.

Many, but not all; have a difficult time switching their basic concepts in stances and simultaneous body movements of the limbs from their old system. Close in the internal, does not always count.

Rather than overcome a student's previous training, it might be better introducing Hsing I power, using whole body power with the step, and origin of force; through the spear. Few have any training in it from before; and no previous training to overcome, is an advantage in this case.

While learning the higher level concepts, introspection is needed to become aware of one's limitations of thinking. Terms of old basic concepts from a previously learned style, must be constantly redefined; otherwise one will never achieve the qualitative level of the newly learned internal concepts and energies. A newly learned arm move, for example, must have the coordinated changes in stances, body mechanics and breathing. If one is unaware of these differences and do not correct related items as you move on, the old way of moving slowly comes back.

After basic movement skills in the long spear are acquired, Five Element Fist can be taught based on the newly acquired methods of the spear's internal foundations.

This spear technique shows how Hsing-i developed the hidden and sliding steps.

When a long enough spear is used (fingertip height), one can be moved by the spear. This is fundamental in chi projection. The longer the pole, the easier to vibrate its tip; however more effort is needed when hands are held close together.

A longer pole compared to a standard pole of six feet, develops chi projection and a more fluid movement of the pole.

Pi Qiang (Splitting Spear)
    I.   Helps with foot transfer in:
        1) forward potential energy and changes in acceleration;
        2) rooting energy and adjustments the ankle/knee/hip wave;
        3) adjusting the blow's direction and projection to a moving root.
    II.   As 'one moves through the forward hand'.
        When one moves through oneself, internal energy is passed through these chambers.
    III.   Moving spear tip up without using arms, by using the torso.

Zuan Qiang (Water Drilling Spear)
    I.   Shows how to pull the body forward, sliding through the front hand; with a balanced reciprocal action.
    II.   One moves forward internally, through inhaling and expanding the body's center.

Beng Qian, (Wood Smashing Spear)
  I.   The rotation of the rear hip forward,
            is coordinated with the hip/shoulder movement,
            in conjunction with the step to provide the thrusting force.
  II.   Does not use the torso or opposite arm movements,
  III.   Teaches the proper attachment to the step, Sacrum, Chi center and
            grounding.
  IV   One may use the same energy by:
            the front sideways ridge hand, low downward block,
            followed by the rear sideways fist hand straight mid-punch.

Pao Qian, (Fire Pounding Spear)
  I.   Rise and twist done in tandem simultaneously by both forward
            moving arms.
  II.   Moving forward from rear cross step,
            transfers to other leg's forward step,
            shaping the spear tip's downward crashing.
  III.   Teaches how to continue a push of your body
            to pull your body along, a fundamental of cloud-stepping.

Heng Qian, (Earth Smashing Spear)
  I.   Forward push of spear, sliding through front arm; and rear leg's
            cross-step forward: coordinated.
  II.   Sliding push of spear through front arm and front leg's advance;
            propels the spear's sideward thrust.
  IV.   Teaches a good reverse T-stance set up,
            for a rear leg roundhouse kick,
            the kick mimicking the later sidewise spear motion.

Hsing-i Five Element Saber

Hsing-i Spear and empty hand should be completed first. Japanese Samurai Sword is based on Hsing-i Saber. A two-handed sword of at least forty inches teaches: blow transfer and focus, arm to arm energy transfer. body to arm then hand jing transfer; coordinating and rooting. Five Element Saber shows scissor-step methods with the rear foot controlling power and root, projected toward the coordinated front foot/ankle, hand/wrist controlling of the martial edge of attack (in this case the saber).

WORKOUTS IN ALTERNATE CLIMATE & CONDITIONS

TRAINING IN THE RAIN WITHOUT GETTING SICK

My basic knowledge consists of breathing through the nose, or a small opening in the mouth, to minimize the moisture/cold shock on the lungs.

For preventative herbs, use garlic, vitamin C, and alfalfa. If it's really bad, use old man's beard, or golden seal, but they should not be taken often.

When not working out at a high activity rate, keeping ginger in the mouth like snuff; will help.

Usually if you are under 30 years old, it is sufficient to work out hard enough, or fast enough to keep one's heat up. An activity rate similar and including jogging is appropriate. When older or lacking sleep; this is not enough, and you can end up getting a bug sometimes, unless the workout is less than 20 minutes.

In doing Hsing-i Metal, in San Ti stance, or on ice, one can:
see where their positioned intention is manifested,
clearly understand their moving root to the ground,
clearly see the root that launches the blow and
clearly feel the root that launches the step forward.

In doing Hsing-i Water, in San Ti stance, or on ice, one can:
focus on first returning to emptiness, then pouring the chi into the rear foot,
clearly feel the root that launches the step forward,
dart the step forward; much like snake or chicken step;
initiate the hand movement from the rear foot-root,
insure that the hand movement springs upward like lightning,
insure that the rear foot remains deeply rooted,
feel the 'bungi chord effect' between the front and rear legs, not quite being shackled.

HSING-I ON SNOW

Training Hsing-i, in the snow, is particularly good for training the focus of the front foot, as it relates to the striking hand.
Although force is usually generated from the rear foot, it is directed and shaped by the front foot. This shaping is more apparent in the snow. Metal is a good one to start with.

WALKING IN THE SNOW

The step could:
stay on top of hard packed snow, or ice,
one could sink to snow depth, or
the step could sink to knee depth or greater.

One should not attach themselves to expecting one depth, or even that the ankle position or bending; will be the same.

The angle of the foot after the fall, relative to the supporting
plane, could be pointing:
uphill/ lifted up
level/ prone or
downhill/ tilted down.

Since the step is dynamic, it is better not to concentrate on form,
or a pre-set way of walking. Every step is different. One should not
just see with their mind or eyes, but with their feet, and center.
The move becomes part of the seeing, not just a result of it!

Qi scientific research at:
http://www.qigonginstitute.org/html/Chen/Waiqianalysis_0704.pdf?PHPSESSID=15f3ab8c81aa134ed7e1acbc3f6e332c

INTERNAL ENERGY WORKOUT

Hard Internal Exercises:

1) Holding the posture **Standing Pole (Embrace the Moon)**, for at least an hour: good for continuous practice, since your energy circuit is circular.
2) Leg press of 4-5 times body weight.
3) V-sit for 2 minutes.
4) Standing in a rooted stance on a train trestle, close to the track, as a train goes by.
5) Sitting **meditations for Chi** circulation: best for concentrating Chi.
6) **Unbendable Arm**; see page 51:
   for learning and testing ability.
7) Holding the **San Ti** posture in the beginning Metal position for up to an hour: best for power in front arm, and foundation for Fa-Jing.
8) Skiing.
9) Surfing.
10) Chinese Spear (page 71), Five Element Spear (page 133), like the long staff will teach moving with the whole body, lower spine and body alignment.
11) Traditional Chinese Long Staff and Iron Pole; like the spear will lengthen the tendons, refine one's fluid step, use flex testing of wave strength, and teach vibrating the tip (Golden Chicken Nods its Head).
12) Iron Pole.
13) Nunchakus (Two Section Staff, Lian Jia Gun {The Sweeper}):
    a) teaches fluid bending action of legs and arm and scissor front step;
    b) develops seeing without the eyes, as the weapon:
       i) is passed behind the back,
       ii) goes faster than you can see and
       iii) is passed behind the shoulder;
    c) OSS and 8 patterns:
       i) for changing direction,
       ii) accelerating,
       iii) orbiting gravitationals,
       iv) stabilizing effect of gyroscopes,
       v) for stepping, as in Ba Gua;
       vi) shows an internally hard (hard and moving with whip action);
       vii) good teacher for rooting and centering if done while walking.

    d) Sweeping action is ideal for catching wide areas; deflecting, blocking and striking: using soft or hard internal energy.

    Patterns of movement lend themselves to quick adjustments of flight path, martial trajectory, speed, focus, potential energy, momentum, and impact area. There are similarities to the gyroscope of effect of riding a bicycle, stabilizing it.

    Others sense similar rotor and/or propeller trends and characteristics. Practice will sweep defects in one's blocking and catching, as well as their moving stance and root. Regular use will sweep away any loose ends in your attire, posture and/or movements.

    Lian Jia Gun is one of the best tools for perfecting blind sweeping catches and awareness. The Golden Sweeper.

14) Three-Section Staff, good for:
    a) throwing yourself into it, and having it throw you;
    b) teaching the coordination of the body's three sections:
        legs, trunk (midsection of chest-abdominal area) and arms.

15) Aido (Samurai Sword Drawing) has origins in Hsing-i Saber:
    a) *scissors step*, a squeezing advancing ground step,
      that is started and driven from the base of the heel section of the foot;
    b) transfer of ground strength to waist, waist to hip/shoulder,
      shoulder to elbow, and elbow to hand;
    c) manifesting internal drawing out of inner energy.

16) Hsing-i Saber, practiced after Hsing-i empty and Spear,
    scissor-stepping and jing focus:
    coordination of rear leg's pedaling the force forward and
    the forward leg's focus of striking tip angle and jing.

17) Bolo Machete,
    axe effect of sword using elbow and full arm, with a fluid step.

18) Bowie Knife:
    axe effect of knife with elbow wrist in fluid full-arm motion.

19) Tomahawk:
    fluid revolving pattern that is directed by the Lower Dan Tien.

20) Battle Axe:
    Directed fluid step, focused by moving root and Lower Dan Tien.
    Teaches use CENTER OF CHI, which is not always the same location as one's center of Chi.

21) Large War Hammer (Thor's Hammer).

TOE TO TOE

You both line up facing each other in a horse stance,
at an agreed distance, that usually starts out at fist length.

This distance is tested on each other's shoulders. The shoulders are used for
a test area only, by all but wimps. Watch or for the collarbone (clavicle), it
breaks with very little pressure.

A non-lethal target is agreed upon, which usually is the abdominal area
above the belt.

A coin is flipped, to decide who goes first. one guy strikes the other, in the
designated area;
under the rule that the striker's feet cannot step, or leave the ground.
Optionally, to further constrict the punch, additional rules:
  no dropping by bending the knees,
  no turning of the hips, or
  no turning of the shoulders.
Then you switch.

If this goes well, the next area to test is the breast plate (sternum), between
the ribs. Best to have some muscle or padding here, some people are not
built for it.   The elderly might no want to risk their more brittle bones. Stiff
people, should avoid this also.   Those who are loose enough, can usually
crack their breast plate and/or collar bone (chiropractic bone reset popping).

If using the chest area for a target, most usually declare the solar plexus out
of bounds. If you are with a trusted partner, and are advanced in Internal
Iron Shirt, you might want to try it. I have had good luck. Even if you
prevent the internal damage in a solar plexus strike, there is danger of that
small triangular bone, snapping, and puncturing something; causing a
hemorrhage. If a wide striking area is used, this usually does not happen.

Soft Internal Exercise:

1) Duck Walk.
2) River wading at a depth of thigh to waist, depending on current.
3) Sinking into the surf sand when the breakers come in,
   to a depth of thighs to waist, watch out for the undertow.
4) Nei Gong: Uniting the Original Chi.
5) Nei Gong: Circling Arms in Front of the Chest.
6) Holding the Hsing-i, San Ti posture in the Metal position,
   for three breaths.
7) Running down railroad tracks in between the rails where the ties are.
8) Running through tires laying flat, as in the football drill.
9) Walking through thickly forested woods, or uneven ground,
   at night without a flashlight, or blindfolded.
10) Carrying a pack of 50-100% of body weight for hours,
   with a vertical rise of 1,000-3,000 feet per day.
11) Nei Gong; Jade Dragon Weaves its Tail.
12) Cliff or ice wall climbing;
13) Ba Gua energy circle walk Single Changing Palm; building the center.
14) Ba Gua energy circle walk Carry the Ball,
   to Lion Opens His Big Mouth; building the center.
15) Ba Gua energy circle walk, Carrying Two Glasses of Water;
   negative energy expelled out and away from the center,
   positive energy built in center.
16) Prayer Hands Chi Sau.
17) Tai Chi Sword.

You need to have eye sharp, hands quick, your step strong, along with 'guts' and overall strength.

EYES SHARP

Ability to detect and "read" an opponent's movements immediately.
Ability to feel an opponent's movements and react accordingly, as in Tai Chi Push-Hands practice.

Hang a small object (like a washer) by a string. The string can be held either by the hand at arm's length or suspended from the ceiling. As you swing the object back and force, following its movement closely with your eyes. Continued practice will strengthen your eye muscles and prevent fatigue. The result will be quicker and more accurate eyes movements.

The second method requires no equipment. Turn your head quickly and focus your eyes on a particular spot you have chosen on the wall. Strive to focus quickly on a small point rather than a large area. This technique further enhances quick and accurate eye movements.

Follow the movements in your forms with your eyes in the direction you are attacking or defending. Focus on strikes and the direction you are moving in. Train yourself not to blink while someone claps in front of your face or delivers a strike just short of the face or head.

Fearlessness, intestinal fortitude or "guts"
Many people have difficulty sparring since they acquire the habit of retreating in defense or after they deliver an attack. Fear leads to hesitation and improper distancing that would be to your disadvantage. Movements must always be quick, aggressive and decisive.

Sand Bag training is best used for general conditioning of the body, strengthening the joints and ligaments to prevent injury from the shock of striking something heavy or immovable. Sawdust filled bags are too soft.

Use at least a 60 pound sandbag.

Sandbag training for power kicks, would be divided into:
 1) kicks that will sway the bag left-to-right,
    using the pivoting motion of the foot knees and hips
    (spinning sidekicks and roundhouses)
    {best to distinguish kicks that:
       start from dead stop,
       continue the pendulum swing, and
       attack the pendulum swing to at least a dead stop}-
       good movement;

2) thrust kicks such as a front, side or back, that go directly forward –
   good linear bag movement, as well as collapsibility of bag;
   structural alignment and impact testing of striking area and body/ground
   connection;
3) vertical and angular kicks –
   only partially manifested by bag movement, but good for testing
   counter reaction to one's stance and grounding;
4) externally hard, shattering, snapping kicks, -
   some bag movement, impact testing of striking area and body/ground
   connection;
5) penetrating kicks -
   will not move the bag, but will test resilience of joints with
   a good soft thud, being the best indicator.

Sandbags can be an excellent test of one's ability to throw multiple punches that are forged by real life situations. Many with 'good form' will find their arm strikes lacking due to weak wrists, and bones that are not used to load bearing or impact. In the ring, boxers tape their wrists.

Although penetration of a sandbag is unlikely with bare hands it is a good test of one's finger strength for spear hands. Many use the sandbag for grappling strength. Finger point strikes can be tested for internal finger strength and trueness of martial trajectory.

Best to increase the calcium in the diet for the bone hammering, lecithin and silicon for the joints.

Watch out for bone bruises. Training should have periods between for the rebuilding of tissue. Remember not to overdue it, since the repeated damage of any area is a breeding ground for cancer.

I have not found the commercial large heavy bags filled with sawdust of be of any use, except for children. A makeshift bag can be made with a marine or Cordura duffle bag, sail canvas, or tent material.

Many people that have not been in fights before, will find their arm's useless after a few volleys with a hard blocking opponent, or limp after being numbed by the impact of their own strike hitting hard bone.

While it might be overboard to train with the sandbag all the time, a disciplined use will forge one's bones, joints, and connective tissues. Striking the bag is a good indicator of flaws, even when it is not the best test for all of the strike's strength.

.-.-.

The best ways to train for "quick hands" is to practice the forms with speed and focused power, after the set has been learned well and practiced enough to eliminate any hesitation caused by trying to remember the next movements. Speed by itself won't get you very far, since the power must also be generated quickly and accurately. Delivery of power needs to be quick. Use speed and power together in a balanced combination to ensure effective execution of technique.

A quick step is essential to closing the gap, or adjusting the distance between you and your opponent for an attack or defensive maneuver

Train single stances for strength. Hold a particular stance, such as a horse stance or bow stance.

Once strength is established, practice moving in and out, closing the gap; then retreating quickly after several attacks have been made. Quickness of stances and footwork are best trained by form practice, since light steps and strong stances are requirement for good forms.

A strong person needs to maintain that strength then learn to focus, then control that strength.

BUSHWHACKING PUSH HANDS

A dynamic method of Push Hands, is to use tree branches as Wooden Dummies, to practice sparring techniques. When one pushes on a green-live limb, it will push back relative to its size, the angle you push at, and the force exerted. If a branch is stronger, it will either remain stationary, or push you back. This forces a good rooting by the practitioner.

If the tree limb is dead, and not to large, it will break, being good practice for external blows, and redirecting internal blows. Once the branch has broken, it is a good sharp cutting object, to practice sweeps on.

The tree and branches are good for practicing covers (a deflected strike that blocks, all at the same time).

Stationary limbs are also good for grabbing techniques, pulling oneself in closer for a strike, or pushing off and spinning to flank.

Do at night, or blindfolded to develop your lower Dan Tien's seeing ability.

At a higher level, one charges through thickly forested woods, bushwhacking their way, and going with the flow. One might trip, but that is all part of the training, since this will help train deflection and rolling techniques. This can also be done at night, but protective glasses are recommended.

This training; emphasizes general principles of moving and internal energy. It does not use static and pre-set methods. This causes one not to use pre-conditioned responses, but to see with their Lower Dan Tien, and their hands.

In the internal, the energy is the same whether blocking or striking, it changes to suite the environment, like water flowing.

For hard style breaking, dead trees in various stages of decay, are good practice, since they additionally check your rooting and balance. Open-handed cutting and piercing strikes may likewise be tested on dead wood, and partially burnt wood.

DYNAMIC BLOCK-STRIKES, COVERS (JOUSTING)

This is an advanced method incorporating a dynamic blocking strike. If an arm is firmed externally, muscles are tensed; it slows the movement and interrupts the flow of Qi.

It is important for the arm to maintain a firmness, while moving, which is done with the same method developed in:
   a. holding the San Ti posture,
   b. holding Embrace the Moon,
   c. Unbendable Arm (page 51),
   d. Traditional Chinese Long Staff
   e. Tai Chi Long Sword.

If an arm is firmed externally, muscles are tensed, which slows the move and interrupts the flow of Qi.

If an arm is firmed by muscle tension, the block's direction is changed, and in physics terms, a loss of velocity results. Losses of velocity equate to a slower speed and less potential power. This negative effect is compounded by the ricocheted effect of the block being deflected, no matter how small. Internally, this does not occur with dynamic block-striking.

COVER PRACTICE

Both practicing partners stand face to face in a relaxed horse stance, at about arm's length distance.

INSIDE-TO-OUTSIDE MIDDLE BLOCK/STRIKE (HORSE)

Partner A will strike toward partner B on his left side with a right handed front punch at the pectoral muscles. This punch should not be pulled, but not have full power either. It does not take much to crack a rib, so be careful.

Partner B will intercept the thrown fist just past the wrist with an inside to outside block that contacts at Partner B's thumb side of the wrist below the hand, then slides as it turns inside. This contact area slides up along Partner A's thrown inner arm as it turns to a palm downward front punch.

This is called a cover, or a block-strike with the same hand; both hand movements of Horse are carried out by the same hand; the inner-to-outward Earth block changing into a mid-height front punch.

The contact area must have resistance or Partner A's fist will slide through. If this resistance is external, it will be rigid, slow and break contact. Use Unbendable Arm (page 51) energy to maintain a fullness in the contact area. The contact area of Partner B's blocking hand will slide as well as the contact area on Partner A's striking arm.

Some have success by seeing Partner B thinking of striking through Partner A's initial strike. This is done by proficient sword fighters. Sliding up or around an opponent's blade, is faster than going around it. Banging swords together is for Hollywood, not an experienced warrior. This eliminates the effect of martial checkers, responding move for move. This does not fight the force it deflects the force by being precise and dynamic.

See with your arm and Lower Dan Tien, do not rely on your eyes.

OUTSIDE-TO-INSIDE MIDDLE BLOCK/STRIKE

Partner A will strike toward partner B on his left side with a right handed front punch at the pectoral muscles. This punch should not be pulled, but not have full power either. It does not take much to crack a rib, so be careful.

Partner B will intercept the thrown fist just past the wrist with an outside-to-inside block that contacts at Partner B's little finger ridge hand side of the wrist below the hand, then slides as it turns inside. This contact area slides up along Partner A's thrown outer arm as it turns to a palm downward front punch.

UPWARD HIGH BLOCK/STRIKE (FIRE)

Partner A will strike toward partner B on his left side with a right handed front punch at the jaw or middle of the forehead. This punch should not be pulled, but not have full power either. To be safest, use the front of the forehead that is used for breaking bricks, stay away from the side points such as those near the temple above the eyes. Experienced contact fighters might want to use the jaw, but this is risky, since some have 'glass jaws'.

Partner B will intercept the thrown fist just past the wrist with an upward Fire block that diagonally contacts at Partner B's little finger ridge hand side of the wrist below the hand, then slides without turning. This contact area slides along Partner A's inside lower striking arm as it turns to a palm downward front punch. applying upward resistance as it slides into the home target base.

DOWNWARD LOW BLOCK/STRIKE (SNAKE)

Partner A will strike toward partner B on his left side with a right handed front low punch at lower intestines. This punch should not be pulled, but not have full power either

Partner B will intercept the thrown fist just past the wrist with a downward inside-to-outside downward block that contacts at Partner B's thumb side of the wrist above the hand, then slides low inside. This contact area slides up along Partner A's thrown inner arm as it turns to a palm downward low front punch, or if block goes down farther, then Snake strike up.

MARTIAL DODGE BALL (SLOCUM)

One person is in the center of a circle, with others lining the outer area of the circumference of the circle.

The people lining the outside of the circle have a dodge ball and throw it at the person in the center. They must stay outside of the circle, or replace the center person when they violate the boundary.

The person in the center stays there, or anywhere inside the circle; till he catches the ball. The center person is freed and whoever threw the caught ball, now replaces the targeted person, in the center of the circle.

When beginning, you might want to regulate the target area so that the head and below the knees are not allowed. A beach ball or whiffle-ball could be used also. Increasing the circle sized will make it easier for the center person to catch the ball and avoid getting hit.

When one wants to toughen it up, try it blindfolded, with a basketball or medicine ball.

KICKS

To do a side kick, use a thrust kick, rather than a snap kick. In both cases the knee is tucked first.

Shotokan does a Side-Snap-Kick,
that is whipped primarily from the knee which is external.

Old style Mo Duk Kwan does a Side-Thrust-Kick,
originating from the Lower Dan Tien;
can be both internal and external, sometimes simultaneously.

All Tai Chi, and Hsing-i are Side-Thrust-Kicks,
are internal only.

FIGHTING

Grapplers are very vulnerable to Dim Mak points and knee attacks; before after and during a throw; more the points after and during a throw, knee attacks before and during for a throw. One who is skilled in falling should not be hurt by the fall.

A take down (trip, slam or assisted yank), is too quick do anything about during or after; only before. Elbow strikes can be effective.

The duration of a throw, on the other hand, is usually much longer than a vital strike.

Leg sweeps are good before, as they prevent the shifting of a grappler's weight before a throw.

QUICK HAND TEST

One classic test for external breaking quickness, is for a partner to lightly hold a 2 inch breaking board at the top suspended by the index finger and the thumb, then you break it. If you are just strong or fast, the board will move and not break. One who has quick hard fist, can cripple an open hand.

A quick kicker can also damage any open hand, but very few are this quick. They will do 1,000 kicks per training session, at least three times a week. Many kickers of average speed, will have their leg trapped by a grappler, and will either be thrown, or have their leg crippled.

An Internal Martial Artist has even more options.

 If the opponent doesn't move, you must be still. If the opponent moves just a little, quickly attack, faster than he. The hand must be flexible and sharp. The step must be light. Forward, backward and turning you must be light, like a cat. If one thing moves, everything must move.

When sparring, you should use both hands to protect the center line at all times. Be careful of attacks from left and right angles. If a punch comes from a straight line, you should cross the bloc. If a punch comes from across, go straight in. (If, however, you are too late to go in, go straight back - regardless of whether the cross-attack is high or low.)

When fighting, either attacking or defending, you must have three points together. Nose, toes and fingers (or fist) must point in the same direction. Use timing and opportunity.

When a punch comes, do not just block; punch back at the same time. That means punch and block together. If you just block, the opponent will continue to attack. That is why you must use the timing and opportunity for attack to keep the opponent busy with defense. The idea is block and hit, control and hit at the same time. That will make you fast, him slow.

No matter what development method you use, you must follow what the classics say: "do not develop part of your body." If you do, later all the movements will lose their harmony. Mind, Qi, breathing, and power cannot be separated or you will lose your power.

Overall Internal Strength

Some key elements for sparring were listed: eyes, guts, quick hands, strong stance/quick steps, and overall strength.
This will deal with overall internal strength and strong stance.

Hard Internal Strength as in blocks, Hsing-i and a fixed stance, Soft Internal Strength as in Tai Chi, Chin Na and a moving stance.

An old classic adage says to learn a new Martial Arts move properly, one must practice it correctly for 1,000-10,000 times. Part of this training involves repetition of the basic move, from a fixed angel, at a fixed distance. A number of repetitions must be at various angles also.

Once solo practice is accomplished, the move must be incorporated for different ground conditions, fighting distance, and counters from the opponent. Many will train with a 'sure fire move' endorsed by the instructor, and assume that it will work under all conditions. This is a laboratory based philosophy without practical applications in the field.

When one trains for multiple variations in martial counters of a move, they are much closer to adapting to the real. Multiple variations can metamorphize the common in all, the universal concept. This essence is experienced, rather than thought, or analyzed. This can be augmented by meditation.

When we were young, my brother and I would get our kicks jumping off a sand bank, onto a 40-50 foot alder tree. The tree would bend from the forward momentum and eventually tip toward the ground near the sand beach, and we could jump from there. When we jumped forward, things did not always go as planned, and we devised a methodology for alternates, as we worked our way to greater heights.

Some of the factors affecting our tree grabbing were: how our hand slid onto to the branch we were catching, how the branch would bend, and how the tree would move forward with our jump from the high sand bank. A moving, and live wooden dummy.

Even this training was not complete, for we had to plan for 2-4 different succession of branch grabs. We would visualize our alternatives before jumping, but his was not enough either. If something went wrong, the next 1-2 alternatives had to be automatic, so they had to be practiced repeatedly also. When the practice was complete, it had to be mentally rehearsed before we leaped, to be fresh enough for success.

The same is true of practicing moves; defensively and offensively. Commercial schools will practice one counter to a move, to build confidence. It is not practical assuming people with different back grounds and body builds will use the same the technique or manifest it in one manner only.

Practicing moves with different responses gives a more rounded view of options, which can develop a feel for which way to go.

Grab the right, enter the left. Grab the left, enter the right. While stepping forward, the heels touch the ground first. The tip of the foot uses the toes to grab the ground.

Before exchanging hands, the Qi is already forward.

When you sense an opening in your opponent while he is calm and postures are ordered; beware, it could be a trap. If your opponent's hands are rising his legs have to be rooted, so he cannot kick effectively. When kicking the root is weak, so the hands are not in a good position to strike effectively.

When rising, expect falling; when falling expect rising. In general, if an attack comes from a side; intercept with the same hand.

When far use kicks, medium range use fists, and when short use elbows, knees hip and head.

Control the opponent's knees to check their kicks,
control the opponent's elbows to check and shape his punches.

Use from two through five-steps blindfolded sparring drills, starting at a slower speed; will give a good martial sense of position.

Nunchakus are good for becoming familiar with the arm movement patterns and passing of power, three sectional staff demonstrates the three parts of the body; arms, torso and legs.

When one becomes proficient enough to go faster than you can see, nunchakus are good practice for catching and blocking.

Nunchaku snaps hitting vertically with the length of the two section staff have some unique properties:
1) as all other weapons hit horizontally with this area as in a club, the 9 section staff hits horizontally with the point, but more in a ball and chain fashion;
2) because of the shorter swing radius and larger mass (staff diameter) of some 2 section staffs (short nunchakus or chucks), a turbine effect can have a balancing effect beyond a pendulum swing. with major gravitational effects.

How do you know that the forms and drills you are practicing; are martially effective?

Is your Qi nothing more than a warm feeling or a graceful flow? How do you know if your internal sets are functional and nothing more than healthy ballet?

The only truly objective test for an internal blow, is by having a soft material such as a four inch thick phone book placed over the abdominal area of a volunteer, who will feel the strike through the material. Beginners should not do this anywhere near the heart, liver or kidneys. If severe internal damage were to occur, the intestines are long, and have a lot of redundancy. It is unlikely that one would feel this on the shoulder, since only hard bone is beneath then immediate surface. Only use a full flat fist or palm, finger strikes might have unintended acupuncture effects.

Start the test with minimal strength, then proceed to ½ strength. The person getting hit should be the more advanced, at least in the beginning. It is imperative that repeated or advanced training be done with Internal Iron Shirt methods such as Golden Bell and/or Cotton Belly.

If the strike is mainly felt on the surface, it is still an external blow. If you are just moved back, it is no more than a shove. A flexible material is used to avoid the billiard ball effect. Do this from two to four inches away, so as to avoid any potential energy that is just accumulated by momentum.

HERBS

Some prefer the caffeine in coffee and colas, for helping alertness, but I do not, since it makes me a little shaky, especially Columbian coffee. If I use caffeine, I usually prefer the green teas.

Yohimbe bark, is even stronger than the Colombian, for those that prefer it. Constituents: Ajmaline, corynantheine, corynanthene, quebrachin, tannins, yohimbine. High doses of yohimbe may cause confusion and disorientation.

Gotu Kola tea, or extract, is generally preferred for sparring or competition. Gotu kola contains triterpene which may help to maintain healthy collagen, which is found in the skin, connective tissue and ligaments. In addition they help to promote healthy blood vessels and may help balance the activity of neurotransmitters, the chemical messengers in the brain.
Some will augment this with caffeine.

JOINT HEALTH

Glucosamine chondroitin nourishes cartilage and connective tissues maintaining integrity of joints, assists in wound healing, strengthens collagen fibers, and reduces pain from osteoarthritis.

Liquid lecithin is good for joint lubrication.

Silicates for the ligaments, between the muscle and joint, they are found in bamboo shoots, okra, horsetail and oatstraw tea.

Gotu kola (Centella asiatica) has been used as a medicinal herb for thousands of years in China, India, and Indonesia. Its ability to heal wounds, improve mental clarity, and treat skin conditions such as leprosy and psoriasis were important reasons for its extensive use in these countries. Gotu kola is used for disorders that cause connective tissue swelling, such as scleroderma, psoriatic arthritis (arthritis occurring in conjunction with psoriasis), ankylosing spondylitis (arthritis of the spine), rheumatoid arthritis, depression, and to improve memory and concentration. Recent studies show applications for gotu kola, treating venous insufficiency (pooling of blood in the veins, usually in the legs), boosting memory and intelligence, easing anxiety, and speeding wound healing.

Stretching, and circular use of each joint in each direction; will also relieve stress, and poor alignment.

Cod liver oil helps relax and strengthen the joints when used daily. It also helps reduce the popping noises of the joints. Apply externally.

For remedial action, massage the area to the bone, with strong fingers, or a piece of polished jade, quartz, or wood.

For those skilled: slight traction, for the popping effect of re-alignment, as in chiropractry.

BONES

Added calcium is critical for:
 the added stress of strenuous training,
 structural impact breaking strength of bones,
 repair of bones,
 bone density and
 any one over thirty.

A calcium supplement is usually best absorbed at night, with food, and augmented with magnesium, vitamin A and D.

Turnips, milk products are rich in calcium. Hamburger usually contains up to 10 % finely ground bovine bone, so it is rich in calcium bearing bone meal. Since oyster shells are brittle, their supplementals are not recommended.

Long cooking stews with bones in them are highly recommended.

Studies have shown that children must have some red meat protein in their diet also for developing bone length mass. Patterns of short limbed children in complete protein diets from different cultures and geography, improved when diets of developing children were enriched with red meat. This was the case in Mexican red bean and corn diet, as well as an Asian rice and soy diet.

For bone strength, there is question whether it is better to eat meat from a large animal such as a cow; or a small low bone density animal such as a bird.

Load bearing exercise keep up the bone mass such as weight lifting, and carrying a pack.

Stimulants, processed sugars and caffeine decrease bone mass and make the bones brittle. They have a negative effect on peripheral vision, accident rates, resistance and objectivity.

Nettles contain many minerals, a tea or spinach of cooked nettles strengthens the bones.

INTERNAL ENERGY

Red panex ginseng will help the flow of Chi, but should not be taken when sick, or with vitamin C. It could be taken before an intense workout. This is a hot, male, and yang herb. Ginseng is a good body warmer. Women should avoid it, but if taken should take the white ginseng. Ginseng contains also contains zinc.

Deer antler (pantochrin), penis and tail, are all good energy tonics, as well as effective for endurance and memory.

Gecko lizard tail prescriptions and kidney nourishing pills are very good, but can give one a hair trigger when taken with caffeine. This should be avoided by those with weak hearts, touchy stomachs, or high blood pressure.

HSING-I FOUNDER
MARSHAL YUE, FEI

The Song Dynasty (960-1280 A.D.) in China was a sorrowful time for the Chinese. Wars with the northern barbarians (the Jin race or Mongolian), corruption in business and government, and starvation were the state of the country.

These admirable qualities were noticed by a certain man in the town called Zhou, Tong. Zhou, Tong himself was a scholar and a very good martial artist who had studied in the Shaolin Temple. Seeing that Yue, Fei possessed many noble qualities, Zhou, Tong began to teach him martial arts. Martial arts as it was taught to Yue, Fei was a complete system involving barehanded combat, weapons, military tactics, horsemanship, archery, and other related subjects.

When Yue, Fei was 19 old, he joined the Song army in its war against the Jin, a nomadic people who had invaded the Northern Song. The Song Dynasty, which was originally located in northern China, had to move to the south to re-establish itself with a new capital and emperor because the Jin had sacked their old capital and captured their emperor. The Song Dynasty which was invaded is known as the Northern Song (960-1127 A. D.), while the Song Dynasty that established itself in the South after the Jin invasion is known as the Southern Song (1127-1280 A.D.. For years the weakened Southern Song had to pay tribute to the Jin to keep them from attacking further south. When Yue, Fei joined the army, the Southern Song was trying to regain its lost land by war.

Yue, Fei became the commander or marshal of the army that was assigned to fight the Jin. Upon assuming command, he instituted a systematic training program in martial arts for his soldiers. Although some martial training had previously existed, Yue, Fei was the first to introduce Martial Arts into the army as a basic requirement before combat. Many times a young man joined the army only to find himself in battle the very next day. After a while, Yue's troops, known as Yue Jia Jun (Yue Family Troop) became a highly efficient and successful fighting unit.

The success of Yue's troops can be basically attributed to three things. First, he made all his training strict; the troops were trained in a serious and professional manner. The soldiers were pushed until they excelled in martial arts. Second, Yue, Fei set up a military organization that was efficient and well run. Third, and most importantly, Yue, Fei created for his troops two new styles of martial arts. The first style which he taught to the troops came from his internal training, and led to the creation of Xingyiquan. The second style, which he created out of external martial arts, was Eagle Claw, a style which put a major emphasis on Qin Na. The external style, because it was learned more easily, and because it had immediately practical techniques, made Yue's troops successful in battle.

When Yue, Fei went into battle, his highly trained troops had many victories as they began to march north. But Yue, Fei had not yet encountered the Jin commander Wu Zhu, who himself had never lost a battle. Wu Zhu's terrifying success was largely due to his main weapon, the feared Guai Zi Ma. The Guai Zi Ma was an ancient version of the tank. It was a chariot carrying armored men, drawn by three fully armored horses which were connected by a chain. It was extremely difficult to disable either the horses or the riders, and so they completely dominated the battlefield.

Yue, Fei found that the horses were not protected in one place, their legs; putting armor on the horses' legs would have made them immobile. It was too difficult to attack the horses' legs with conventional arrows and spears, so Yue, Fei devised two simple but effective weapons: a sword with a hooked end, which was extremely sharp on the inside edge of the hook, and a shield made out of a vine called "rattan" (Teng). This army was called Teng Pai Jun, or "The Rattan Shield Army."

The Rattan Shield Army crouched very low in the path of the Guai Zi Ma. Before the chariots could reach the soldiers, they ran into obstacles such as upright spears and ditches; which Yue, Fei had had set up. As the slowed chariots advanced, the crouching men; hooked and cut the legs of the horses: making them fall. The shields were greased so the horses slipped every time they put their feet on them. They only had to cripple one animal to stop a chariot. Once a chariot was stopped, other soldiers surrounded it and killed the riders.

Yue, Fei then went north, regaining lost territory and defeating such Jin generals as the Tiger King and Great Dragon. The Jin leaders successfully bribed one of the most infamous men in Chinese history; Qin, Kuai to stop Yue, Fei. Qin, Kuai was at that time the prime minister, and the most influential man at the emperor's corrupt court.

While Yue, Fei's army moved north, Qin, Kuai, sent an imperial order with the emperor's official golden seal (Jin Pai), asking Yue, Fei to come back. According to tradition, a general fighting on the front line has the option of refusing an order to retreat. Qin, Kuai was counting on Yue, Fei's patriotic sense of loyalty to the emperor, sent 12 gold-sealed orders in one day; so much pressure made Yue, Fei return.

When Yue, Fei returned; he was imprisoned. Since Qin, Kuai feared that any sort of trial would reveal Yue, Fei's innocence, he ordered an officer named He, Zhu attempt to find some excuse for imprisonment, but he found nothing. He, Zhu found that Yue, Fei had lived a spartan life, and had fewer possessions than a peasant . When He, Zhu returned to Qin, Kuai, only reported that at the time Yue, Fei joined the army, his mother tattooed: "be loyal and pure to serve your country" (Jing Zhong Bao Guo), on his back.

With such an honest general as Yue, Fei, Qin, Kuai had only one alternative-to have his food poisoned. Yue, Fei died in jail on January 27, 1142 A.D. Yue, Fei was thirty-eight years old. Later, Yue, Fei's adopted son, Yue, Yun, and Yue, Fei's top assistant, Zhang, Xian, were also killed.

For twenty years Yue, Fei was officially considered a criminal. In 1166 A.D., the new emperor Xiao Zong refused to believe in the treachery of Yue, Fei, and relocated his grave to the beautiful West Lake (Xi Hu) in Hangzhou. In front of the grave are stone statues of Qin, Kuai and his wife, kneeling in repentance and shame before Yue, Fei. Emperor Xiao Zong bestowed upon Yue, Fei a new name which symbolized what he always was and always will be: Yue Wu Mu Yue, the righteous and respectable warrior.

JI LONG FENG

Legend has it that Xin Yi Liu He Quan was complied by Yue Fei, and was written down in his Quan Pu, boxing manual. The manual was lost for many centuries until it was discovered in the hollowed truck of a tree.

Ji Long Feng (1588-1662 AD), a former solider of the Ming Dynasty; developed Xin Yi. During the new Qing Dynasty, many former Ming Dynasty military went into hiding to plot the overthrow of the new rulers. Ji LongFeng was one of them. Ji Long Feng was well known for his skill with the long spear. He went to the country seeking recruiting people to join for the rebellion. The Qing rulers were not considered Chinese as they were from Manchuria.

Ji Long Feng was well known and would carry his spear wherever he went A Taoist monk approached him, and seeing the spear knew immediately that it was Ji Long Feng. The monk asked, why do you always carry a spear around, why can't you use the same spear techniques for empty hand boxing?

Ji Long Feng thought about this in seclusion for several days to think about the monk's question. From this question, Ji Long Feng developed Xin Yi Liu He Quan; Mind Intent Six Harmony Boxing.

The harmonies are External Harmonies and Internal Harmonies.

External Harmonies
 hand and foot;
 shoulder and hip;
 elbow and knee.

Internal Harmonies
 mind and intention;
 intention and qi;
 qi and strength.

Xing Yi History and Ji Long Feng

Ji Long Feng may well have learned the old Taoist's Neigong (internal exercises) and Shenfa (body methods) for Soft Hands and Six Harmony Spear.

After learning the Shenfa of Six Harmony Spear, Ji practiced day and night on the banks of the Yellow River, eventually gaining the level of Six Harmony Divine Spear. He then set off again for Shaolin temple.

By this time, Ji took the route, over the mountains and across the Yellow River to the Three Gorges. He passed the provincial seat of Henan and arrived at Shaolin. Ji's horse lost its footing and fell into the valley below. Ji scaled the tall cliffs to safety, relying on his kungfu.

During the days while he spent searching for a route to climb up, Ji watched the local birds and animals and gained an understanding of 10 animals, and more inspiration for the style he was to create.

Although one can learn some fundamentals of animal movement while climbing a cliff, it is unlikely that Ji created Hsing Yi Animals, based on this. More likely they were the product of a long term development not finalized till the 1800s.

Hsing Yi's Five Element Spear and Five Element Fists are very similar, so it can be seen how the empty hand evolved from Ji's spear methods, but not the Hsing Yi Animals.

Ji's "Six Harmony Spear" skill was incomparable, and the abbot at Shaolin Si begged Ji to stay at the temple to teach. In the Shaolin temple's archives, there is a spear manual titled, "Teacher Ji's Spear Manual" (Shi Yong Wen, originally from Shaolin, still has it).

The manual in question is exactly the same as the "Xin Yi Liu He Chang" manual. From this, we can see that Shaolin treated Ji respectfully and called him Ji Lao Shi (teacher, Ji). Not just the manual, but also the tablet erected in honor of Ancestor Ji by Shaolin previously. It was seen by a Ji family 17th generation descendant during the first few years of the Republic (ROC). However, it was destroyed during the military invasion of Shaolin.

Ji's effect on Shaolin can be easily seen. Ji's grand disciple, Li Yi Ming of Henan, struck up a friendship with Shaolin's abbot around the years of the emperors' Yong Zheng and Qian Long's reigns. Li presented the abbot with a copy of the manual "Ten Principle Theories of Xin Yi Liu He", written by him in the 11th year of Yong Zheng's reign. It was treasured by generations of Shaolin monks.

The 12 moves Xin Yi Liu He (Shaolin Xin Yi Ba) as passed to the abbot by Li, were taught only to monks of abbot level. It's a pity that Shaolin has gone through so much trouble, that those who still know Xin Yi Ba's 12 moves are almost gone and the 12 moves are totally different from their original appearance.

Ji, on returning to Jun village, thought of how he should defend himself now, since peace was now here, and swords and spears were no longer carried. He thus modified his spear style into an empty hand style, using the intricate shenfa of the 13 posture Soft Hands (the 5 bows of the body) and added the 10 animals, creating Xin Yi Liu He Chuan; the principal "when moving the path cannot be seen, once moving is effective."

During the Ming Dynasty, one famous for Six Harmony Spear Li Ke Fu, who used Mei Hua Liu He Chang (Pear Blossom Six Harmony Spear).

The treatise written by Chen Zong You in 1621, "The Selection of Long Spear Ways", details the style he learned from Li. General, Qi Ji Guang, who lived in the same era as Li, had gone to Tang Jing Zhou, 21 years his senior, in search of instruction, and it is possible that he had asked Li, who was the same age as him, for instruction too.

In his "New Book of Effective Techniques" are records of Yang Family Spear's "8 Mother Spears", "Six Harmony Spear" and "24 Spears". The Six Harmony Spear in Tang's book, "Martial Edited Selections", has little differences with the Six Harmony Spear recorded in Qi's manual.

Yang spear's "Six Harmony Spear," also known as the "Plum Blossom", or the "Plum Blossom Six Harmony Spear", is related neither to the Yang Spear of the Yang warriors of the Song Dynasty, nor to the "Plum Blossom Spear" of Yang Miaozhen (the wife Li Quan leader of the Red Coat Army).

The latter is the combination of a spear with a tube of flammable substance in front, lit before battle, with the aim of burning one's opponents; "Flames and the spear thrusts".

Liu He Spear was known from the Ming Dynasty onwards. By the Year of Wan Li, Henan's Li Ke Fu was already very famous. Wang Zong Yue was also of this period. Taoist Dong of Qian Zhai may, just like Cheng Zong You, have been taught by Li Ke Fu.

The names of forms in Xing Yi Spear and Wu Taiji are similar. Chang style, that came from Wang Bao Spear; also has 13 Spears, 21 Spears and 24 Spears etc, and also includes 3 point theory, similar to Xin Yi Liu He. In 1887, Mai Zhuangtu's disciple Ding Zhao Xiang visited Chang Nai Zhou's hometown to converse with his 5th generation descendant Chang De Pu, he made a copy of Chang Nai Zhou's treatise, "Tendon Change Classic, Chi Channeling Secret", and included it in his boxing manual.

The 13 postures, which originated from Taoism, have an undeniable relationship with Xing Yi.

Chang Nai Zhou (1724-1763) wrote the "Central Chi Theory", and the twenty or so chapters on the "Theory on Yin Yang Entering and supporting" were called the "Tendon Change Classic, Chi Channeling Secret." The 3 Point theory contained within seem to be from the same source as the 3 Point Theory in the Xin Yi Liu He boxing manual. This may be due to the fact that Chang was a student of Wang Bao Spear, which came from Taoist Dong of Qian Zhai Temple.

Taoist Dong had incredible skill with Liu He Spear and Staff, and was also an expert in the Taiji 13 Postures. Taoist Dong was an old man when Ji LongFeng was around 30, could it be that Ji gained his Liu He Spear and Staff from Dong?

Chang Nai Zhou had a friendship with Chen Village's 12th generation descendant Chen Ju Xia and his "Tendon Change Classic, Chi Channeling Secret" may have been passed to the Chen Village at that point.

One of Chang's teachers was "Holy Taoist Yan of Luoyang". At this point in time, at this very place, Henan's Li Yi Ming's "Ten Principle Theories." were copied by Ma Zhen Ding and Wang Zhen Lin, active during the years of Qian Long's reign. Perhaps they passed a copy to Taoist Yan, who passed a copy to Chang, and Chang passed this, along with his treatise, to Chen Village?

Chen Family 16 generation descendant Chen Xin once used Taiji theory to edit the Xing Yi Boxing Manual. The part he edited being "3 verses on 10"(translated, 3 verses about 10 principles/theories?) and renamed the manual the "3, 3 Boxing Manual"(trans. 3*3=9).

The 14th generation descendant Chen Chang Xing also modified a copy of Xing Yi's "9 Theories" which was passed into Wen county into "Chen Taiji Theories".

Another of Chang's teachers was Taiji Master Li He Lin, and from the boxing style Chang created. He learned from Li He Lin was the "Taiji Health Maintaining Skill" created by Li Zhong, Li Rui, and Chen WangTing, or Tongbei.

Otherwise, there would be no need for him to create a new style, and also, there has been no copy of the Xing Yi Boxing Manual found in Bo'Ai county.

Zhaobao He style disciple He Youlu's 'Manual of He Style Taijiquan,' in the second appendix, Chen Ji's manual from 1804 and Chen Xin's book, written at eighty years old in 1928, not only relate the direct relationship between the boxing and weapons fighting of the Chen family and the Tongbei gong of Qianzhai Temple (Tongbei Reeling Boxing/Tongbei chanquan) and the origins of Paochui. They also explain why Chen Xin, in his book 'Explanation of Chen Family Taijiquan,' took the word 'reeling' as the soul of Chen Taiji. They confirmed that Chen Xin's 'Three-three Boxing manual' was a combination of the Xinyi Liuhe Manual, Yijin jing's 'Formula of Connected Harmonies' and the Tongbei Reeling Boxing Manual.

People believed that 'Three-three' was a reference to Xinyi Liuhequan but when compared to a few of Xinyi Liuhe manuals with the table of contents to Chen Xin's 'Three-three Boxing Manual'; there were a few inconsistencies. The 'Yijin jing Formula of Connected Harmonies' , came from Naizhou's writings. This means that those uncertain parts of Chen Ji's and Chen Xin's books were from the Tongbei gong manual (Tongbei Reeling Boxing) of Qianzai Temple. Thus, Chen Xin combined the Xinyi Liuhe Manual, Yijin jing's 'Formula of Connected Harmonies' and the Tongbei Reeling Boxing Manual together in his book, calling it the "Three-three Boxing Manual.' The fact that it came from these three sources explains the significance of the word "three" in the title.

During an earlier study of Taijiquan's history, quoted from Du Yuanhua's book 'Orthodox Taiji,' which said that Jiang Fa's teacher Old Wang was from Taigu in Shanxi. It also made use of Zhaobao Taiji practitioner Zhang Jingzhi's writings, which were passed down to Yang Bangtai and then to Huan Dahai, stating that Jiang Fa's teacher was "Wang Zongyue from Shanxi, Seven-Mile Village in Jinyang."

Some questionable sources were used above. There is no 'Seven-Mile Village' (Qili bao) in Jinyang or in Taigu. Moreover, Taiyuan and Taigu are very far away from Bo'ai County in Henan (Originally HeneiCounty) and Zhaobao Village in Wen County. If Wang Zongyue was a traveling merchant from Shanxi (in pre-modern times, Shanxi was called Shanyou (Right of the mountains) and Shandong, to the east of the Taihang mountains, was called Shanzuo (Left of the mountains), to travel from the Taiyuan or Taigu areas to Henan seems like a very long journey, which is suspicious.

In Chen Xin's manuscript, between the 'Explanation of Spear and Pole' and the 'Four Sets of Hammers' is the chapter 'On Differences in Boxing.' The Qing dynasty Fenchuan Prefecture is modern-day Xiangfen County, Hefen County and Yicheng County (in Shanxi). In Yicheng County there is a Wang Village which in the Qing was known as Lesser Wang Village.

Lesser Wang Village was old Wang Zongyue's hometown!

From Wang Village to Yangcheng County in Shanxi and the border with Bo'ai County in Henan it is just a short distance. If Wang Zongyue were to go to Henan on business, this would be the only possible route. Because of this, it is perfectly reasonable to suspect that Wang passed by Qianzai Temple, where he passed on his "13 Soft hands" to the Daoist Dong Bingqian. He also passed through Zhaobao Village, only 40km from Bo'ai (there was a Shanxi Hall there in pre-modern times), where he encountered Jiang Fa, mourning his parents' death, and took Jiang Fa with him back to Wang Village in Shanxi where he taught him the "13 Postures Boxing."

Xinyiquan was created by Ji Longfeng based on his understanding of natural principles, his virtuosity in Six Harmony Spear and the methods of the Thirteen Postures, and a thorough understanding of Tongbei Reeling Boxing. Completely breaking away from the massive content of Tongbei Reeling Boxing's 108 postures (known as the 'source of all boxing'), returning to the root from which all those variations sprang, Ji took the most simple and essential aspects and boldly created his own boxing style, softened the Tongbei Reeling Boxing and created the 'Taiji Life-Nourishing Exercises.'

These exercises still retain the traditional movements and postures of Tongbei Reeling Boxing.

Ji's 'Discussion of Spear Methods' and the Tongbei Reeling Boxing 'Discussion of Six Harmony Spear Methods' have many similarities. However, Ji's discussion is much more refined and innovative; this is due to Ji's extraordinary cleverness and thorough understanding.

Because of these qualities, Ji reached a different level than his fellow student of the Qianzai Temple's martial arts, Wang Zhongjin of Wang Village. This can be seen by comparing Ji's writings with the 'Wang Village Spear Manual.'

In Tongbei Reeling Boxing, there are '72 Grabbing and Seizings,' '36 Coiling Throws,' '37 Rolling Throws,' and the word 'reeling' is considered to be their highest secret. In Xing Yi Quan there is no grabbing and throwing.

In the Xinyiquan formula, there is 'moving heavily, moving lightly, and finally moving nimbly.' In the 'Internal Power' chapter of the 'Discussion of Ten Important Points,' 'sticking jin' is listed as the highest form of internal power, saying that it can 'eclipse the sun and moon.'

In Tongbei Reeling Boxing's 'Battle Methods,' it says, 'Advance from the side; dodge quickly and win with clever [technique].' Xinyiquan also has 'Contract the body and advance from the side like a tiger pouncing on a sheep; as soon as one shot has hit the mark, the troops should implement a clever strategy.'

Tongbei Reeling Boxing has 'When the hands strike and the feet do not follow, [the attack] is 90% empty,' and 'At a distance, use the hands; close-up, use the elbows; when you are neither close nor far, use leverage.' This is practically identical to Xinyiquan theory.

All in all, the Qianzai Temple in Bo'ai, Henan and the Zhongnan Mountains are in opposite directions from Ji's hometown of Yongji; Ji would not have gone all the way to Zhongnan Mountains.

The above loosely based on Steven Yan's paper, Ji Long Feng (Xin Yi History). What Ji Longfeng considered when creating his new style, March 2007.

Nobody really knows what the real link between Yue Fei is, and Hsing Yi. The book that is said to be written by him is in question by some martial art historians. Currently there is no direct link that Yue Fei is the starting point of Hsing Yi so many historians say that the history starts with Ji Long Feng. Some historians believe Ji created Hsing Yi based on the spear and his previous knowledge of Shaolin.

Many styles based their history on a famous hero to attract attention to their particular style, i.e., based on Yue Fei knowledge of Shaolin, he created Hsing Yi and Eagle Claw. Some say: if you study Yue Fei's Bio, you'll notice that he never had time to develop any style at all because he was too busy being in the army, fighting the enemies of China and always running to one battle to another. It could be asked, when did he really have time to create anything?

A martial art is tested by battle, and in this regard, Yue Fei is a very practical inventor of Hsing Yi.

The principles that Yue Fei used in his own martial skills were the bases of Hsing Yi so that is why many people give him as the creator of Hsing Yi.

There is no connection between Hsing I and Shaolin Temple. It appears that Hsing-i develop outside of Shaolin. The burning of Shaolin temple had no direct effect on Hsing-i except to drive it, like all other styles, underground when teaching to others.

This Hsing-i came from Sun Lu Tang who learned the Hopei style of Hsing-i. SLT then used principle of Bagua and combined the principles of Hsing-i to develop his own unique style of Hsing-i in the early 1920's and as some historians have labeled Sun Lu Tang's Hsing-i as a sub branch of Hopei's style.

None of the BSL lineage from Yim Chi Wen on back learned Hsing-i. They were only masters of BSL as in those days; knowledge of any kind of martial arts was a trade and was not shared or easily learned from anyone.

It was the Boxer Rebellion that made people aware that their style will die if it was not taught quickly, to a wide range of people. People did not want to learn martial arts anymore as it was no longer a trade or skill needed to make a living as a security guard in an escort business. Trains and motorized vehicles replaced the escort business. With that said, KYC was lucky to have learned Hsing-i from SLT because he was at the right place at the right time when SLT came to visit Li Ching Lin when KYC was learning Tai Chi and Wu Tang sword from Li.

MARSHMALLOW GUT (COTTON BELLY)

WANG SHU-CHIN

A student of the famed Chang Chao-tung on the mainland, Wang's Hsing-i and Pa-kua were orthodox, and machined to perfection. With his bulk, hands the size of small rosebushes, and his surprising speed, the goal of Hsing-i-to occupy the enemies territory-was adroitly done. The internal system stresses the cultivation of chi, deep breathing, and a drastically different approach to the mechanical aspects of fighting ... . like Shao-lin it has many advocates who can withstand with impunity a foot or fist to the midriff. Wang not only has this skill, but can actually use his vast stomach against one's fist on impact so as to produce a broken wrist. Throughout Asia he has been tested , and no one comes close to hurting him. Leading Japanese karate masters have bowed to him after failing on his punch.

But this alone cannot make a fighter. Frank "Cannonball" Richards, the carnival performer, and various other "marshmallow gut" types in the United States have the capability to take a stomach attack. Indeed, Harry Houdini died as a result of his inability with this feat. After ineffectually Wang's belly once, I asked if he could take a solar plexus strike. "Try it," he said. I did-several times, with no effect. But beyond this special skill Wang could do something beyond the ability of all the fighters I saw. He could take any kick to the lower extremities(excluding, of course the groin). I kicked him repeatedly on his knee, calf, and ankle until my feet ached, all with no effect.

" How do you do it?" I asked.
His answer: "Chi."

Such skills do not connote anything more than defensive ability. Coupled in Wang, these skills left an attacker only two targets, the head and groin, both very mobile and difficult to hit. But one still might properly ask, could he fight?

He could and did. He has spent much of his time in recent years in Japan and has fought several high-ranking karate men. No one has come close to defeating this seventy-year-old warrior. In the process he has come to a supreme depreciation of karate. He feels that the original forms borrowed from China have been distorted and that the nonsensical high kicks and vigorous body hardening avail nothing when confronted with real technique.

169

And technique he has. He uses Hsing-i fist with a corkscrew twist from one inch out with more effect than most men get form a full-stance strike. John Bluming, Dutch amateur judo champion and Mas Oyama's prize foreign karateka, even though he had hurt his wrist on Wang's stomach, disparaged him to me once when I was visiting Tokyo. "What else can he do?" asked John. I took John to Wang and asked that he be shown the corkscrew, but to keep it gentle. Wang put his relaxed fingers on Bluming's stomach, curled them into a fist and screwed. Bluming bent over in agony and has since been a believer.

Chinese Boxing, Masters and Methods, by Robert W. Smith, pages 72-74, published by North Atlantic Books, Berkeley, CA, 1974, 1990

CANNONBALL RICHARDS

Footage of Cannonball Richards showed the enormous man take a cannonball right in his mighty abdominals, only staggering back a foot or two, followed by a piece called "Edge" in which STREB performers whammed themselves frontally against a wall of Plexiglas placed between them and the audience

From: Seattle Union Record

RECOMMENDED READINGS and LINKS

Chinese Boxing, Masters & Methods, by Robert Smith

Xing Yi Quan Xue, The Study of Mind-Form Boxing by Sun Lu Tang

Qigong, the Secret of Youth, Dr. Yang Jwing-Ming's YMAA Publications, YMAA Publications

XingYiquan, Theory, Applications, fighting Tactics and Spirit: by Liang, Shou-Yu & Dr. Yang, Jwing-Ming.

Chinese Mind-Boxing, by Robert Smith, Advise From the Masters, by Kuo Yun-Shen

Hsing-I: Chinese Mind-Body Boxing by Robert Smith, from Kodansha Press in Japan (1981, **ISBN 0-87011-476-X**, but his new book called Hsing **Yi**, with his student is not recommended, due to its external focus.
Good reprinting recently: Hsing-**I** book title, now Hsing-i: Chinese Mind-Body Boxing, originally **ISBN 1-55643-455-3** by North Atlantic Books.

Classical Xingyi Quan Vol 111, Xingyi Mu Quan (Mother Fist) by Jiang Rongqiao (1929), translated by Joseph Crandell (1999),
Smiling Tiger Martial Arts, Pinole, CA, 94564.
This is an excellent translation by Joseph. He learned from Peter Ralston who learned from Grandmaster Wong Jack Man.

Xing Yi Nei Gong by Dan Miller and Tim Cartwell 1994,
High View Publishing, Pacific Grove ISBN 1-883175-04-6.
This book is known for securing and transmitting information from old Hsing-I manuals and collecting in one volume. This is not a direct lineage to our style of Hsing-I.

The Handbook of Alternatives to Chemical Medicine, by Mildred Jackson, and Terri Teague; out of print: yet available.

The Art of War, by Sun Tsu

Flatland by Edwin Abbot

Sphereland, by Burger

Tai Chi: Tai Chi Touchstones, Yang Family Secrets, by Wiley Publications or Wayfarer Publications.

Any of the books on Phenomenology: by Martin Heidegger or Edmund Husserl.

Dim-Mak Death Point Striking, Erle Montaigue, Paladin Press.

Animals in Translation, by Temple Grandin PhD.

There are many manifestations and signs of Qi, but these are not Qi. When one is full of Qi they are powerful and energetic, when low in Qi, one is tired and/or sick, when out of Qi – your dead.

People can lift cars in an emergency by using Qi. Naysayers say this is because of the adrenalin. It might be argued that the muscles have moiré power with Qi, but only Qi will strengthen the bones to allow the lift, without the bones breaking.

A competent teacher is a student's best mirror and hope of focus. This book will help. It teaches how to feel Qi, not eye-based visualization. Sensing-seeing is done with your gut (Lower Dan Tien), hands, feet etc. Training is individually based and free of the limitations of different languages, religion, or culture; since ones own experience is utilized to learn to recognize previously felt sensations of positive and negative Qi. The 'Shared Lived Experience' and essences are the means of communication, and development. This eliminates the extra step of translation.

Qigong is based on meditative martial Northern Shaolin Buddhist methods, Internal Iron Shirt and Internal Iron Palm in the Wide Circle of Kung Fu of Joseph Greenstein (The Might Atom of Ripley's and Guinness Book of World Records. Hsing-i was studied under Grandmaster Wong Jack (Chia) Man of San Francisco Jing Mo (the first person to complete all of the Northern Shaolin studies since World War II). Sifu Wong's direct lineage can be traced to the Ching soldiers burning of Honan Shaolin Temple 1732 AD., when Monk Chi Yuan escaped and went to Shantung province. Sifu Hayes has taught Hsing-i, Shaolin, Tai Chi and Qigong at: the Yoga Den (Rainforest Yoga), in Juneau from 1991-1998; Juneau Public School's Community Schools, from 1991-2005; private lessons in Juneau, since 1995.

ISBN 978-0-578-09972-9